CW00556148

The First Book You Need to Read
About Low-Sugar Life
for the Entire Family in 5 Simplified Steps.

SUGAR DETOX FOR

BUSY MOMS

Discover How to Lose Weight Now

as a "Side Effect" of Sugar Detoxification.

Olena Sieger

© **Copyright 2022 - All rights reserved.**

The content contained within this book may not be reproduced, duplicated, or transmitted without direct written permission from the author or the publisher.

Under no circumstances will any blame or legal responsibility be held against the publisher, or author, for any damages, reparation, or monetary loss due to the information contained within this book, either directly or indirectly.

Legal Notice:

This book is copyright protected. It is only for personal use. You cannot amend, distribute, sell, use, quote, or paraphrase any part, or the content within this book, without the author or publisher's permission.

Disclaimer Notice:

Please note that the information contained within this document is for educational and entertainment purposes only. All effort has been executed to present accurate, up-to-date, reliable, complete information. No warranties of any kind are declared or implied. Readers acknowledge that the author is not rendering legal, financial, medical, or professional advice. The content within this book has been derived from various sources. Please consult a licensed professional before attempting any techniques outlined in this book.

By reading this document, the reader agrees that under no circumstances is the author responsible for any losses, direct or indirect, that are incurred due to the use of the information in this document, including, but not limited to, errors, omissions, or inaccuracies.

CONTENTS

Thank You!

Thank you for choosing a healthier life!
Thank you for buying this book!
Thank you for trusting me, a busy mom, just like you!

A free gift just for You!
5 Weird Morning Rituals
That Will Help You to Lose Weight.

Discover the "Missing Ingredient"
in Weight Loss Programs.

Scan the QR code below:

Or visit this link:
www.olenasieger.com/5-weird-morning-rituals-to-lose-weight

INTRODUCTION

Would you like to stop your sugar cravings and help your entire family eat less sugar? But at the same time, still enjoy special occasions like vacations, birthdays, holidays, and get back on track? Then you need to keep reading…

Being a mom is a big responsibility. But for the moment, we will focus just on eating habits. Your family depends on what you buy and what you cook. As a mom, you have these little humans relying on you for everything they need, and I haven't mentioned partners who are also counting on you! Plus, a partner might be like a kid too… As a result, you are so focused on your family you often forget to feed yourself properly.

Does this sound familiar? It's almost lunchtime, and you haven't eaten yet, or it's nearly midnight, and you still have a big "to do" list? Your energy is low, and you search for ways to perk yourself up. Usually, the first thing that pops up in your mind is "food". Most of the time, it is easily accessible food that does not require cooking. And this is how poor eating habits start forming.

My life completely changed when my 2 kids were born. Of course, I had plenty of moments of joy. At the same time, I needed to adjust to a new routine with much less sleep. I needed to manage a full-time job, family, and stress every morning while taking my crying kid to daycare. In addition, I was learning something new every day about handling different situations with my kids.

I was fighting with my depression and discovered that eating something sugary made me feel better. Of course, it was a "fix" in the short term, but I did not realize this initially. I was busy with other stuff. It was so comfortable to eat something sugary and feel satisfied and energetic. That is why I continued to do this repeatedly for so long.

I kept relying on sugar until I realized that my kids were copying me. They often ate a granola bar or cookies because they thought it was a good snack. After all, Mom always does it. This realization was like an electric shock for me. Only then I realized that taking care of myself is the same as taking care of my entire family. And if I got addicted to sugar, my family eventually would be as well. I needed to prevent this. And I started with myself to be an excellent example for my kids.

My goal is to eliminate the control sugar has over me. But at the same time, I wish to have the ability to celebrate holidays with my family. I cannot imagine Christmas, Easter, or Halloween without sweets. When kids are around, candies, chocolate and cookies are around too. In addition, I cannot imagine my family without fresh fruits (fruits are also a source of sugar). Discovering a way to reduce processed (not natural) sugar from the family menu is challenging but rewarding because I am not aiming to be completely sugar-free.

So, I started my research about sugar detox by reading books and even enrolled in a few courses. I received plenty of helpful information, but frustrations came along the way as well.

One of the biggest frustrations was when I paid money but received a meal plan for just one month. I cannot say that the meal plan itself was bad, but it just wasn't for me. Some of the food in the plan wasn't food I eat, some I couldn't find in local grocery stores, and other food was very expensive. And there was no guide on how to replace food that did not work for me.

Another frustration was that I needed to cook for myself separately from the rest of my family. Introducing a lot of new meals and rules to kids is challenging. It takes more time for them to realize why we should do things in a new way.

The subsequent frustration is the suggested use of supplements, pills, and powders. Again, the program itself was nice, but I got tired of seeing promotions for supplements. Every time I logged into the application, I would see annoying ads that I couldn't turn off. The supplements might do a good job, but it just wasn't for me and not for my family. I believe that everything my body requires can be found in nature, and there is no need to put lab-produced items into my body. In addition, supplements are not for every budget.

My final frustration is the length of the sugar detox plans I looked into. On the market, you can find programs where participants reported impressive results. But the question that was never answered was, "What do I do when the program is finished?". Most probable, gradually, you will go back to your starting point. While the program might work, I don't know how to maintain my results.

Even with those and many other disappointments, I did not give up because I knew it was impossible to write a book or create a course that would fit everyone. Instead, I continued my research and filtered information from the standpoint of a busy mom with a family. With my research in hand, I decided to put all this into the book "Sugar Detox for Busy Moms" and share it with moms just like me. Here are a few examples of what is covered in this book:

- You will discover the "missing ingredient" that will skyrocket your success with sugar detox,
- We will address one of the biggest challenges that people are facing during sugar detox - how to stop sugar cravings,
- A family-oriented plan with no need to cook separately for yourself, and tips for kids,
- Explanations regarding what to do after detox and how to come back on track after the holidays,
- No use or promotions of supplements, pills, or powders, and a budget-friendly approach,

- This is not a cookbook with recipes. If you are interested in a recipe exchange, I will invite you to join our free Facebook group:

https://www.facebook.com/groups/weight.loss.for. busy.mom

- References to multiple scientific research articles and journals are explained in a simple way,

… and much more.

What about a "personalized approach"?

"Sugar Detox for Busy Moms" covers the main principles and methods you will apply to YOUR current menu. You will be working with YOUR shopping list, gradually improving it at YOUR speed. And if you are open to something new, you can adopt my suggestions about a specific food. If you like it, keep it. If not, skip it.

In addition, you are welcome to join our Facebook group already mentioned above. You will receive support from others going through the same journey in this group. Many have similar challenges, and we help and support each other by sharing experiences, tips, hacks, and some laughs.

And remember, you are mom and sugar detox is just the next thing you have to figure out. And a weight loss will be a pleasant "side effect" of sugar detoxification.

Let's do it together!

1

STEP 1 - EDUCATE YOURSELF

B efore we begin the actual sugar detox process, we need to educate ourselves. Sure, you could go to the Internet and spend days and weeks researching how to be successful at detoxing from sugar, eliminating cravings, and then trying to figure out how to make it all work for your life as a busy mom. That's not necessary because I've already done all of that. As I mentioned in the introduction, I started this process for myself - I knew that the promise of being "fixed" in 21 days wasn't reasonable. I wanted something sustainable that would consider that detoxing from sugar isn't the only thing happening in my life. As exceptional multi-taskers, we need a plan for success.

WHY SUGAR IS THE #1 REASON YOU'RE GAINING AND CAN'T LOSE WEIGHT

The average American's daily *added* sugar intake is 22 teaspoons (Harvard School of Public Health, 2013). (Please, note that this statistic is subject to change.) The biggest contributors to this excess of sugar intake are sugar-sweetened beverages and breakfast cereals. The American Heart Association recommends a drastic reduction in sugar intake because of the frightening obesity and heart disease epidemics (American Heart Association Inc., 2019). I know this information is specific to the United States, but the statistics are very similar when you look into the sugar intake of other developed countries. Just like me, you are motivated and want to overcome reliance on sugar and eventually lose weight. To understand why sugar is such a huge culprit in weight gain, we need to cover how our body and brain respond to sugar. In addition, we will have a look into food marketing tricks that "force" us to eat more sugary stuff and some tools that will help us make better food decisions.

The Body's Response to Sugar

It's important to understand what happens to and within our bodies as we tackle our dependence on sugar.

Glucose is a simple sugar obtained through the food we eat (mainly sugar and starches), and it is easily converted to energy. It is also essentially the sole source of energy for our brain. Because the neurons in our brain cannot store glucose, they require a constant stream to function appropriately. Insulin transfers glucose from our blood to the brain and muscles to be used as energy (Smith, 2020).

However, our body needs just a limited amount of fuel (glucose). Any excess beyond what can be used immediately must be stored for later, and when our bodies keep the excess, the fuel is transformed into its "storage form" (called glycogen). When necessary, the liver can convert glycogen back to glucose. Once our bodies have over about a day's worth of glycogen, and there is still extra glucose hanging around in our blood (from what we've eaten or drunk), our liver starts turning glucose into fat. The issue with this is how our body chooses where to get its energy from, and unfortunately, our bodies always choose glucose, not fat. Meaning that if you constantly have glucose or glycogen (from overeating sugar), your body will use it for energy and leave the fat right where it is. Insulin is the hormone that is in charge of handling glucose. Insulin prevents your body from using the fat over the glucose or glycogen stores. In comparison, if we eat less sugar, it means that our body will eventually deplete the excess glycogen. Less blood sugar means lower insulin levels, which forces our bodies to use fat as energy rather than using glucose or converting glycogen to glucose (Smith, 2020).

Summary: When we eat sugar, glucose or glycogen are present in our body. That leads to the presence of insulin as well. And insulin does not allow our body to use fat as fuel. As a result, we are getting fatter.

The Brain's Response to Sugar

A part of our brain functions as a "reward centre" called the limbic region. It is responsible for a number of positive responses, from satisfaction to euphoria when part of it is stimulated. On the other hand, it is also responsible for reactions like fear and pain when other areas are stimulated, called the "punishment centre". Experiments have shown that if an experience does not produce a response in either of these centres, it is very unlikely to be stored in our memory (Mad'a, 2016).

Similarly, if an experience indeed does create a reward, like eating sugar-laden products as a way to gain energy, our brain stores this information. This action and response are then reinforced for future situations where we have a sense of needing to feel "better" (Mad'a, 2016).

Summary: When we eat sugar, we stimulate our brain's "reward center". And we store in our memory that sugar is a way to gain energy. The brain will release signals of sugar cravings every time we have low energy. And we get addicted to sugar.

"When we eat sweet foods the brain's reward system — called the mesolimbic dopamine system — gets activated. Dopamine is a brain chemical released by neurons and can signal that an event was positive. When the reward system fires, it reinforces behaviours — making it more likely for us to carry out these actions again. Dopamine "hits" from eating sugar promote rapid learning to preferentially find more of these foods (Reichelt, 2019)."

"So what happens in the brain when we excessively consume sugar? Can sugar rewire the brain? The brain continuously remodels and rewires itself through a process called neuroplasticity. This rewiring can happen in the reward system. Repeated activation of the reward pathway by drugs or by eating lots of sugary foods causes the brain to adapt to frequent stimulation, leading to a sort of tolerance. In the case of sweet foods, this means we need to eat more to get the same rewarding feeling — a classic feature of addiction (Reichelt, 2019)."

So many of us (myself included) reach for something sugary to get through particularly tough parts of our days. As we learned, sugar affects the part of our brain that responds to stress and can make us believe we are less stressed out. But this is actually suppressing our brain's ability to respond to stress appropriately, thus causing a reliance on sugar to properly process stressful situations (rather than using our inherent skills). So not only have we tricked our brains into thinking that we are less stressed-out, but we're also going to get fatter while we do so because we're consuming sugar-laden food to do so.

Now you understand why it is important to take care of our bodies and brains. Until science figures out how to do a full-body or brain transplant, we only get one of each during our time on this earth 😊

Summary: Sugar changes chemicals in the "reward center," leading to suppressing our brain's ability to respond to different situations appropriately.

Until we "re-program" our brain to receive "reward" from different things (not from sugar), we are going to get fatter because we are consuming sugar-laden food.

THE FOOD MARKETING TRICKS

We just learned that we "program" our brain to eat more and more sugar in different situations. But we will not stop there. Let us see how food manufacturers get into our brains as well.

Companies that sell highly processed sugary foods have absolute marketing geniuses working for them. Did you ever notice that apple farmers do not spend a ton of money on advertising during big sporting events? Did you ever wonder why?

It's simple - nobody is disputing that apples are good for us. There are no research studies, parent coalitions, or mom social media groups trying to make us more aware of the potentially harmful effects of fresh fruit.

But when something is inherently bad for us, it needs convincing marketing. The absolute worst part of this marketing is the intense focus on appealing to children. This is one reason why this book acknowledges that as busy moms, we can't (and don't) live in a bubble that excludes our families. In a later chapter, we discuss how to bring our children along with us as we remove our reliance on sugar.

Food and beverage companies that sell high-sugar products have big marketing budgets and spend billions of dollars each year on advertising. Soda pop and other sweetened beverage companies top the list with over one billion in yearly marketing spending. Other types of companies with huge advertising budgets include sugary cereals, baked goods, snack foods, and less-suspicious foods like bread, soup, yogurt, and salad dressing (Union of Concerned Scientists, 2016).

While these companies do not outright lie to us as consumers, research performed by the Union of Concerned Scientists (2016) has shown the tactics used can be very deceptive. For example, they may take a lower-sugar food and advertise the higher-sugar version as a new flavour or with more appealing addi-tions. Another tactic is to use words like "fruit", which sounds healthy, but it may mean they've added sugars to mimic fruit flavours, without the benefit of actual fruit.

Also, did you know that you are a target of sugary-food marketing as a woman? The Union of Concerned Scientists (2016) has shown that we are targeted through gender-based messages as women. This specific marketing strategy is based on traditional family roles. And we, as women, are targeted because in the majority of families, we are responsible for groceries and cooking.

We may not have even realized that these companies were getting into our brains. Good thing we are strong, competent, and taking things into our own hands and making the changes to better ourselves. We got this. And with this awareness, we will work toward a healthier lifestyle.

Summary: Fresh fruits and vegetables do not need advertising. In contrast, big food manufactures are spending big budgets on ads. Their marketing geniuses target kids and women and try to convince us to buy sugary food. Be aware of that and take responsibility into your own hands.

GLYCEMIC INDEX

Now, when you are aware of sugar's effects on the body and brain, you probably wonder which food to decrease or avoid to prevent sugar spikes in the blood. We will now discover some tools that will help us answer this question.

An essential tool in determining how quickly food makes glucose enter the blood is called the glycemic index (GI); it is a rating system for food (1 – 100; low – high). Sugar (pure glucose) is rated at 100. On the Internet, you might also find GI calculated using white bread as the reference food instead of glucose (Foster-Powell et al., 2002). But in our book, we will use GI that was calculated with glucose as the reference food.

The Glycemic Index is classified into 3 groups:

Low Glycemic Index (GI): 0 to 55
Moderate Glycemic Index (GI): 56 to 69
High Glycemic Index (GI): 70 and over

The Glycemic index of the most common food can be found in Appendix 2.

Food that causes the blood sugar levels to increase dramatically (or spike), such as candy, soda pop, or cake, is rated high on the glycemic index. Studies show that food with a high Glycemic Index has lower satiating effects, leads to hunger and stimulates eating (Foster-Powell et al., 2002). Food with a slower release of sugar, resulting in a more consistent bodily response, such as most fruit and vegetables, and dairy products are rated low. The lower the food on the glycemic index, the slower our body processes and digests it, and this is usually because of the fibre in the food.

If you take a deeper look at tables of the Glycemic Index on the Internet, you will note that values vary for different food brands or even for the same type of food. And many factors affect GI. Here are just some of them: ingredients, processed method, cooking time, testing methods, the accuracy of measurements, the location where food was produced. Rice is one example of a food that needs to be tested by brand and location. Also, you might note that **some food like salad vegetables, cheese, eggs, avocados, fish, meat, and poultry are not included in tables with the Glycemic Index**. And the reason for that is the very little amount of carbohydrates in this food (Foster-Powell et al., 2002). **It is safe to consume them for a low-sugar lifestyle.**

We provided the list of Glycemic Indexes in this book to give you an idea about what type of food belongs to what type of GI.

Summary: Glycemic Index (GI) is a rating system for food based on its effect on blood sugar levels. For a low-sugar lifestyle, it is safe to consume food with low GI (0-55), sometimes acceptable food with moderate GI (56-69), and we need to work on decreasing or completely removing (if possible) food with a high GI (70+).

Salad vegetables, cheese, eggs, avocados, fish, meat, and poultry are not included in tables with the Glycemic Index because they contain little amount of carbohydrates. It is safe to consume them for a low-sugar lifestyle.

GLYCEMIC LOAD

Now that we understand Glycemic Index (GI), let's go one step further - Glycemic Load (GL). GI does not consider the portion size or grams we need to eat. This is where the GL becomes very handy; GL is a more comprehensive measure of the effects of sugars in our food. GL is calculated by multiplying GI (with glucose as a reference food) by the amount of carbohydrates in grams per serving size and dividing the total by 100 (Foster-Powell et al., 2002). And tell us how much glucose will go into our blood due to eating that portion of food. This results in a more accurate insight into the food's effect on blood sugar.

According to the 2020 article "Glycemic index diet: What's behind the claims", the University of Sydney classifies Glycemic Load into 3 groups (Mayo Clinic, 2020a):

Low Glycemic load (GL): 0 to 10
Medium Glycemic load (GL): 11 to 19
High Glycemic load (GL): 20 and over

You can find the Glycemic Load of some food in Appendix 2.

It is important to say that the majority of healthy food has a low Glycemic Index. However, there are a few exceptions. For example, you might think that according to GI, you should avoid watermelon (GI = 72). However, watermelon mainly consists of water. And for a reasonable portion (120 grams of watermelon), GL is very low (GL = 4). The same applies to pineapple.

Confused? Don't let this overwhelm you. Maybe some other food has high GI but low GL, but I found just two that we already mentioned above: watermelon and pineapple. The GI is a perfect place to start, and avoiding high GI foods won't lead you astray. There is no food that is low on the GI that suddenly finds hiding sugars or carbohydrates and is high on the GL. The table in Appendix 2 with Glycemic Loads can give you an idea of portion size. Information about GI is easy to obtain, but you now have a deeper understanding of achieving success. Your insight into GL has provided you with a great foundation to detox from sugar!

Summary: Glycemic Load (GL) has more practical value because it considers portion size. Recommendations for a low-sugar lifestyle are the same as for GI.

It is safe to consume food with low GL (0-10), sometimes acceptable food with medium GL (11-19), and we need to work on decreasing or completely removing (if possible) food with high GL (20+).

There are a few exceptions like watermelon (GI = 72, GL = 4 per 120 grams) and pineapple (GI = 66±7, GL = 6 per 120 grams) with high GI but low GL. If you respect portion size (120 grams), it is safe for your low-sugar lifestyle.

DIFFERENT TYPES OF SUGAR - "GOOD" VS "BAD"

I'm going to start this section by saying that, despite this title, I actually don't believe in categorizing foods as "good" or "bad". The psychological impact of these labels can be harmful and misleading. Labelling food in this manner is especially harmful for children, because it can lead to shame/hidden eating, overeating, and other eating disorders. However, because this isn't a book for children, and I'm trying to simplify the complexities of which sugars we should or shouldn't eat, we'll use those labels.

Natural Sugars - Why They're "Good"

Natural sugars occur in food as it was created. Anything that comes out of the ground, off a tree, or existed before us doing anything to it will have natural sugars.

> *"Sugars naturally occurring in fruits, vegetables and dairy are ok but sugars removed from their original source and added to foods, we need to be wary of."*
>
> — (GAMEAU, 2015)

Fructose is the natural sugar found in fruits and vegetables, but once it is removed from these foods and put into other foods, it is no longer a "natural sugar". Another natural sugar is lactose, found in milk and dairy products (Gameau, 2015).

You may think fruit is not sweet enough to help you overcome your reliance on refined sugars. And this is because you trained your body and mind to believe that fake sweet is better than natural sweet. Our society promotes the idea of fake being better than real, and our food is no different when it comes to marketing. But think for a minute about biting into the absolute perfect, dark red strawberry, or a deep yellow and fragrant piece of pineapple. This is how nature intended us to receive our sugar and the satisfaction that goes along with it - without the highs and lows that come with refined sugars.

There's a reason behind the increase in those interested in low or no-sugar lifestyles. In our society, we are starting to recognize just how detrimental refined sugars are to our bodies, minds, and children.

We briefly covered natural sugars previously. I need to make sure, you realize when we're talking about natural sugars that fruit juices aren't included. "Natural sugars" only refer to fruits (or vegetables) in their natural state, as they are in the back of the farmer's truck.

We need to consider the cellular structure of the whole fruit, which contains fibre. Fibre fills you up and keeps you from overeating (Gearing, 2015). Did you ever notice how eating half an apple is much more satisfying (hunger-wise) than a few pieces of chocolate? You can thank fibre for that.

The cellular structure of fruit matters because our body has to break down the cells of the fruit before its sugar can be released into your body. This means the sugar is absorbed into your bloodstream much more slowly, raising your blood sugar levels in a slow and controlled way. This also promotes feelings of being full and prevents overeating (Gearing, 2015). But we can't say the same about chocolate or other sugary, processed food.

Summary: "Natural sugars" only refer to fruits (or vegetables) in their natural state. Fruit juices aren't included. The main difference in "natural sugars" is fibre. Fibre promotes feelings of being full and prevents overeating.

Refined/Added/Processed Sugars - Why They're "Bad"

The American Heart Association defines added sugars as: "any sugars or caloric sweeteners that are added to foods or beverages during processing or preparation. Examples include putting sugar in your coffee or adding sugar to your cereal. Or with food that has sugar already added, sugary prepared coffee drinks or high-sugar cereals. Added sugars (or added sweeteners) can include natural sugars such as white sugar, brown sugar and honey, as well as other caloric sweeteners that are chemically manufactured (such as high fructose corn syrup)." (American Heart Association Inc, 2017)

Before you believe this is an overly simple concept where added sugars are easy to identify, there are at least 60 different terms for added sugars, which I have outlined in Appendix 1 for you to reference easily. To add some simplicity to the concept of the many different ways to identify added sugars, you can remember that any ingredient ending with "ose" is an added sugar (American Heart Association Inc, 2017).

Aside from the list in Appendix 1, it's important to know that sugars are hidden in food not commonly considered "sweet". For example, tomato sauce and ketchup are loaded with sugar. Also, food that is often considered healthy like yogurt, granola, or whole-grain cereals, can have a lot of processed sugar.

In 2016, the Food and Drug Administration changed the Nutrition Facts label to show both "Total Sugars" and "Added Sugars" (American Heart Association Inc, 2017). However, some companies had until January 2021 to switch to include added sugars.

So why are these sugars "bad"? We covered this previously in this Chapter, where we unveiled how sugar affects your body and brain. But I'm more than happy to cover it again briefly, because we're busy moms, and maybe we don't have time to go back to the beginning of this Chapter: "Bad" sugars make us gain weight, cranky, emotionally unstable, more hungry, and can lead to irreversible damage to our bodies.

Summary: Any sugar added to food during processing or preparation is considered "Bad" (refined/added/processed sugar). There are at least 60 different terms for added sugar (see Appendix 1).

Sugars are hidden in food not commonly considered "sweet". For example, tomato sauce, ketchup, yogurt, granola, or whole-grain cereals.

WHAT DO YOU NEED TO KNOW ABOUT ARTIFICIAL SWEETENERS?

Artificial sweeteners are not as they appear - they are not our "get out of jail free" card when we're craving some unhealthy refined sugars. Research on these is still new, and there is currently not enough information to prove that artificial sweeteners are worse than refined sugars like high-fructose corn syrup. However, studies have shown that artificial sweeteners do not reduce and may even increase weight gain over time (Gearing, 2015).

If you compare table sugar with artificial sweeteners only calorie-wise, you might think artificial sweeteners are great alternatives. However, you need to know how those sweeteners affect your brain and body. Consider the following before making your decision regarding artificial sweeteners:

- "These chemicals are **produced in labs and factories** and are not found in nature (Nolin, 2022)."
- "Artificial sweeteners all have different chemical formulas. Some resemble natural sugars while others are radically different. They are usually **many times sweeter than sugar** – saccharin is an incredible 200 to 700 times

sweeter than table sugar – and some of them are hard for the body to break down (Nolin, 2022)."

- "Research has suggested that consuming lots of artificial **sweeteners scrambles the bacteria in our gut**, causing them to make our bodies less tolerant to glucose, the main building-block of sugar (Conner & Brown, 2018)."

- "Consuming sweeteners **change how the body processes fat** and gets its energy at a cellular level (Conner & Brown, 2018)."

- "**The more artificial sweetener you consume, the more fat your body creates** and stores (Chichger, 2018)."

Summary: Replacing processed sugar with artificial sweeteners is not a solution even though they have less calories.

The biggest concern is that artificial sweeteners can change how we taste food. It may cause us to find foods like fruits and especially vegetables less appealing.

READING LABELS - A HOW-TO GUIDE

As we already know, the ingredients listed on a label can be deceiving. The 60 different names for sugar are an excellent example of how we can be fooled into thinking that we are choosing a low-sugar food when it can be laden with sugars.

So beyond the basic ingredients, it's important to know how to read the nutritional tables on the food we purchase. Obviously, these tables are only relevant to processed foods, which are preferable to avoid. But let's be real here - we're busy moms, and we deserve (and need) the ability to feed ourselves and our families things that are easy and require little prep. So we'll cover how to make the best decisions when it comes to this food.

As we know, the American Heart Association has raised red flags about the amount of sugar we eat every day (American Heart Association Inc, 2019). Obesity and heart disease rates are at an all-time high, and refined/ added sugars are a huge culprit.

Recommended Daily Sugar Intake

According to the American Heart Association, recommended amounts of **added** sugar per day are no more than the following:

Women: 25 grams = 6 teaspoons
Men: 36 grams = 9 teaspoons
Children (2-18 years old): 24 grams = 6 teaspoons
(American Heart Association Inc, 2019; American Heart Association Inc, n.d.-b)

Here is a handy approximate formula to remember (Harvard School of Public Health, 2013):

4 grams of sugar = 1 teaspoon

Summary: Above are recommendations for refined/processed/added sugar only. There are no recommendations for "natural sugar". But keep in mind that "natural sugar" occurs only in fresh fruits or vegetables together with fibre. And fibre protects us from overeating. But moderation is a key, even for "natural sugar".

New Label Requirements

A useful thing to remember when it comes to reading and interpreting labels is to avoid food where sugar is the first or second ingredient. On the label, ingredients are listed in descending order by weight. Where sugar lands in the ingredient list is a good indicator of how much sugar that food contains (Harvard School of Public Health, 2013). However, as we have learned, there is a growing list of different kinds of sweeteners.

It is a law that the Nutrition Facts Label lists the grams of sugar in every product on the shelf. But the same food can contain in the same time natural and added sugars. There have been many battles regarding how food and beverage manufacturers have attempted to hide added sugars in their food. Previously, they weren't required to distinguish between naturally occurring and added sugars, but the new label requirements include a line disclosing "added sugars" (U.S. Food & Drug Administration, 2021).

Figure 1 is a sample of the new label from the U.S. Food & Drug Administration (FDA) website:

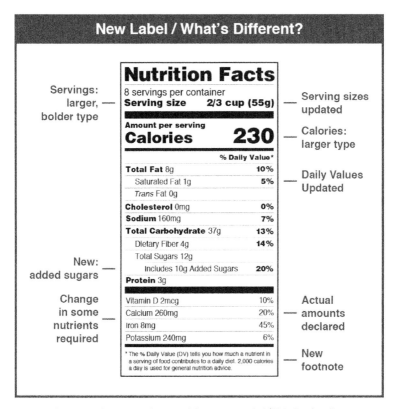

Figure 1. Changes to the Nutrition Facts Label (U.S. Food & Drug Administration, 2021).

The FDA defines "Total Sugars" as including "sugars naturally present in many nutritious foods and beverages, such as sugar in milk and fruit as well as any added sugars that may be present in the product". "Total Sugars" have no "Daily Reference Value" because there is no recommendation for the total amount of Total

Sugars to eat each day (U.S. Food & Drug Administration, 2020a).

The FDA definition of "Added Sugars" is "sugars that are added during the processing of foods (such as sucrose or dextrose), foods packaged as sweeteners (such as table sugar), sugars from syrups and honey, and sugars from concentrated fruit or vegetable juices" (U.S. Food & Drug Administration, 2020a).

Summary: In the old labels, natural and added sugars are represented by one total number. It is still the case in some countries.

In U.S. new label requires "Total Sugars" and "Includes Added Sugars". So, there is a separate number for added sugar that is very handy.

Serving Size

It is important, beyond the ingredients and daily intake percentages on the label to note the serving size. The serving size should be compared to the number of servings in the package, and then will help you determine just how many servings you are consuming. The serving size is listed first in a standard unit, such as cups or pieces, to make it easier to compare with similar foods, followed by a metric amount (U.S. Food & Drug Administration, 2020b).

The serving size is how much an average person typically eats or drinks, but it is not a recommendation of how much we should eat or drink.

Summary: Pay attention that the nutrition label is done per serving size. Serving size is not a recommendation. It is just for your reference and the possibility to calculate actual numbers for the amount you eat.

WHY WE NEED SOME SUGAR

We already discussed how our brains require sugar to function because sugar is the main source of fuel. We do need sugar for our body's optimal functioning.

I just want to highlight that when I'm talking about needed sugar, I'm referring to naturally occurring sugars, not added or refined sugars.

Naturally, sugar occurs in fruits, honey, cane sugar, some root vegetables, and dairy products.

Summary: According to scientific research, natural sugar is required for our body and brain. In the current book, we assumed that natural sugar is fine in moderation, and we are not aiming to be 100% sugar-free.

HOW TO LOSE WEIGHT NATURALLY WITH SUGAR DETOX PLANNING

Everything you need to start and sustain your new life-style is within these pages. I've explained how sugar affects your brain and body. We know how to identify different types of sugars and how they can "hide" in our food. I covered artificial sweeteners and the lie that the food and beverage manufacturers want you to believe about them, and how to read labels to make the best decisions for you and your family. Lastly, we studied why we do need to eat some sugar. Using the information learned throughout the Chapter, we are well equipped to provide our bodies with the "good" sugars.

We'll ensure that you are well prepared, body - mind - and pantry, to start your sugar detox journey. This is infinitely better than jumping into something without the background and preparation to succeed. You have chosen this path because it is important to you, so take the time to prepare accordingly.

The final Chapter in this book will explain how to make your new lifestyle stick. We are starting with confidence, knowledge, and a plan. Our families will see that we are making our (and their) health a priority, and how we've integrated them into our plan.

At the beginning of this Chapter ("The Body's Response to Sugar"), we mentioned that insulin prioritizes glucose over fat as a fuel. However, if we succeed (and we will!) to decrease or eliminate added sugar and eat natural sugar in moderation, there will be insufficient glucose in our blood. Our body will start using fat to get energy. As you can see, with sugar detox you will lose weight naturally.

Summary: Preparation, planning, and main-taining results are essentials for a successful sugar detox.

Weight loss is a "side effect" (in a good sense) of sugar detox because our body starts using existing fat as fuel during detoxification.

So let's continue with mind preparation!

2

STEP 2 - PREPARE YOUR MIND FOR SUCCESS

I n my opinion, **working with your mind is a "missing ingredient" of many sugar detox and weight loss programs**. The power of our minds is more significant than we realize. Our mindset is where our success starts, and where all of our greatest achievements are stored. It's where we draw on our strengths to overcome obstacles, and it's how we will release ourselves from our reliance on sugar. Preparing our minds for success is just as important as preparing our bodies and our surroundings, so this Chapter is the next step in our triumphant journey!

MINDSET

In her article "How to Use the Power of the Mind to Reduce Sugar Intake", Dr. Isabel Serrano is straightforward in her advice: "Stop saying and thinking 'this is hard." When you keep filling your mind with negative and unproductive thoughts, you will start believing them even if you're not predisposed to them (Serrano, 2021).

You Need to Change Your Mind Before You Change Your Lifestyle

A famous and classic children's book called "The Little Engine that Could" has some staying power and wonderful lesson for kids. Perhaps, as a mom, you've read it, but I'll cover the premise of the book.

A train filled with wonderful things breaks down, and cannot move another inch. Trains come by, and the little clown travelling in the train flags them down and asks them to help them and pull the train to their destination. Some of the trains believe themselves too busy or important to take on this task. One train simply believes that he is incapable and chugs off saying "I cannot, I cannot".

Along comes a very small blue train that would never normally be expected to carry this kind of load.

Nobody would expect her to help this long train, but she decides that the plight is important enough that she absolutely must try. She starts by saying "I think I can". She then says this repeatedly until she gets moving, makes it over the mountain, and delivers the contents of the train that broke down (Piper, 2000).

"I think I can. I think I can. I think I can" (Piper, 2000). If I can suggest as much, I highly recommend reading this book with your children. It is an excellent example of being able to do whatever they set their minds to, even when they are very little. The moral of this story is exactly what we are working on here - the power of the mind in overcoming challenges and how if you simply tell yourself that you can do something, it creates a new mindset of believing in yourself which leads to success.

Summary: You and your belief in yourself are the keys to detoxing from sugar.

Why Most Diets Fail

You are going to be the exception to the rule. While the statistics for most diets aren't promising or encouraging, you're not dieting. You're not "quitting sugar", and the process in this book will support you as you reframe how you see and consume sugar, without the huge crash. We consider that you cannot detox from sugar in a bubble, on a tropical island somewhere, surrounded by people who tend to your every need. This process is based on reality. As a fellow mom, I have integrated my new lifestyle into my life and the lives of my family members. Any "diet" or "program" that promises you will completely change your life in a short matter of days or weeks simply doesn't consider most moms.

Dr. Mark Hyman wrote a 2014 article called "5 Reasons Most Diets Fail, and How to Succeed". Here is a summary of the major culprits in the lack of "diet" success:

1. Not backing up your willpower/mindset with science

Simply denying ourselves what we want triggers cravings. Eating certain foods, including sugary foods, actually increase hunger and slows metabolism. One of his key methods to prevent this "failure trigger" is to eat low-glycemic foods with every meal.

2. Calories in and calories out

As we covered previously with the GI/GL, not all calories are created equally. Food that spikes insulin is shifting metabolism. Once again, the way to avoid this is to focus on the quality of food you eat.

3. Not having a plan

Preparing your mind, body, and surroundings is imperative for success. Believing in yourself and having emergency snacks for when your willpower is fading is key!

Summary: Most diets fail because they have "short-term" goals and no plan to maintain results. In addition, during the diet, there is no time to "re-program" your mind for success.

You Cannot Change Your Body Without Changing Your Mindset

Our thoughts are where everything starts, and thoughts generate emotions. These emotions result in us taking action. When we repeat these actions, they become behaviours, and these behaviours become habits (Serrano, 2021).

Based on this, if we tell ourselves "I can do this. I can detox from sugar", we will start to associate a positive emotion with the process. We will begin to feel pride and achievement because we believe in ourselves. Then, because we want to maintain this positive emotional state, our actions will follow, and we will start making decisions that will lead to more positive emotions. As this is reinforced, we have behaviours that become habits, and one day we realize that we haven't craved sugar in a while, and that we've been automatically making healthier decisions. All of this started with our mindset.

Summary: Thoughts, emotions and actions are connected. Actions determine our behaviours and habits. Habits will affect how your body looks. The reverse is also true. When you want to change your body, you need to change your habits, behaviours, actions, emotions and thoughts.

Evening Rituals: If You Want to Start Your Day Well, Finish Your Day Well

One of the best ways to ensure you start your day on the right foot and with a positive mindset is to set yourself up for success the night before. Having a focused, mindful evening allows you to reframe your day and reset your mind, leaving the day behind and looking forward to future possibilities and positive outcomes.

Routines are key to mindset and behaviours, and changing our mindset and behaviours around sugar is essential to overcoming any reliance on it. A simple evening routine gives our minds a bit of reprieve from the challenges that come with our everyday lives. Routines are especially important for children, because their brains are growing and learning, and they have big feelings in little bodies. Knowing exactly what to expect provides a sense of comfort and security, so why not give this to ourselves as well?

Here is a simple evening routine that you may wish to implement:

1. A 30-minute outdoor walk with your children.

Get some fresh air, enjoy each other's company, and spend time looking at the beauty that surrounds you.

2. Before you go to sleep, open the windows in your bedroom.

Flush out the "old air" and create a fresh space to sleep. If you wish, close your window before you go to sleep.

3. Treat yourself.

Take a bath with essential oils or Epsom salts, or relax somewhere quiet and listen to relaxing music. Ensuring that you take some time for self-care means that you have more to give the next day. You can not pour from an empty cup, so filling your cup will allow you to be your best you.

4. Remove your cell phone, tablet, and computer from your bedroom.

The gadget-free bedroom will help you to have a better sleep.

5. Practice visualization.

We will discuss next.

Visualization

Visualization is used by athletes, celebrities, and the more spiritually inclined to achieve success or inner peace. But you may not have thought about applying it to something like detoxing from sugar and living the life that you desire, free from reliance on sugar.

Spending time in this kind of meditative state will create a shift in your mindset. You might not have as many cravings a day, or might not feel like you need to reach for sugar to get through a situation where you normally would. But the effects of visualization are compelling.

In the article "Sports Visualizations" by Keith Randolph, one example of the success of visualization is described. Australian psychologist Alan Richardson experimented with visualization on basketball players. He divided players into 3 groups. Group 1 practiced free shots 20 minutes per day for 20 days. Group 2 only practiced free shots on day 1 and day 20. Group 3 had the same routine as group 2, but in addition, they practiced visualization for 20 minutes per day between days 1 and 20. The results were surprising and terrific: Group 1 improved their results by 24%. Group 2 did not show any improvement. But group 3 improved their results by 23%. With hardly any physical, actual practice, the group that spent 20 minutes a day doing visualization exercises had almost the same results as the group who did the training (Randolph, 2002).

Doing the visualization part of your nightly ritual can look like this:

1. Find a quiet, calm space.

Lie or sit down somewhere comfortably, where your head is supported. You can do this as you're lying in bed.

2. Picture your body as you want it to look, free from reliance on sugar.

Perhaps you want to lose some weight, maybe you want to be fitter, and possibly your body is exactly the same but filled with more energy and the "lightness" that comes without so much sugar. Spend the time to "look" at yourself, and feel how you would feel in this new body.

3. Picture yourself in your daily life, making better choices with what you eat.

If you often rely on sugar at night (like I did), see yourself choosing a better snack, or no snack at all. If you usually drink sugary drinks, picture yourself drinking a cool, refreshing glass of water or some hot, flavourful tea. Take the time to imagine how these better options taste and feel. Feel the crunch of crisp celery or a fresh apple, and how things smell and feel in your hand.

4. Picture your emotional triggers and how you will respond to them without sugar.

See yourself in a stressful work situation, or with children who have a hard time, and imagine yourself doing something other than reaching for a sugary snack to make things better. For example, diving in the swimming pool or just taking a shower and how water removes all stress out of you. Or if you are at work, you go out, find a tree, touch it and let that tree "swallow" all bad energy. See yourself fully recharged.

5. Visualize yourself after you have completed the sugar detox, and feel that sense of pride.

See yourself succeeding on your terms, in a way that makes sense for your life, and setting an excellent example for your children.

Summary: Routines are key to mindset and behaviours. The evening rituals listed above are an excellent starting point for "re-programming" your mind.

SETTING YOUR GOALS

"When it is obvious that the goals cannot be reached, don't adjust the goals, adjust the action steps."

— CONFUCIUS (551-479 B.C.)

Often, individuals plan to change their lifestyle in any manner, but the expectations are pretty lofty, particularly with their eating habits. This can lead to frustration, and often people give up, because it seems the end result isn't achievable. However, as Confucius so cleverly said, the issue is not with the goal. It's how we are working toward the goal that needs to be changed.

Detoxing from sugar is no different; there are many plans and programs that promise big things in a small amount of time. This may be attainable for some, but it wasn't for me. Although detoxing from sugar was a very important thing in my life, it wasn't the only thing, and I needed a plan that would take the realities of my busy mom's life into consideration. I needed to create achievable goals and ensure that my expectations were reasonable.

There is almost a decade of documented research on goal-setting and on the best methods for achieving success. Here is a brief history of some of that research from a 2019 article called "What is Locke's Goal Setting Theory of Motivation?" by Tocino-Smith:

- People who write their goals are 50% more likely to achieve them than those who don't,
- White down your goals,
- Goals that are deliberately outlined, are measurable, and have a concise timeline are more effective,
- Discussing your goals with someone you trust or making them public greatly increases your chances of success,
- Keeping your goals to yourself means they are likely to be lost in the 1,500 thoughts an average person has every minute,
- Achieving a goal usually means giving something up and/or changing habits or beliefs about yourself,

- Setting goals within the framework (a calendar) typically has a success rate of 90%.

Summary: When you start working with your goals, keep in mind the following:

- Do not adjust the goal, adjust the steps to achieve it,

- Write down your goal,

- Share your goal. You are welcome to do it in *our Facebook group "Weight loss for busy moms" (link to it you can find at the end of this book)*,

- Use a calendar.

We will review two theories about goal setting: Vroom's Expectancy Theory and Locke's Theory of Goal-Setting and Motivation.

Expectancy Theory

Vroom's Expectancy Theory suggests it is the expected results that motivate our behaviours. For example, your willingness to detox from sugar is worth it because of the rewards of a healthier lifestyle. The actions you take on your sugar detox path are based on whether you expect to happen (healthier lifestyle, healthier body, healthier mind) actually do happen (Williams, n.d.).

Expectancy Theory has three components: expectancy, instrumentality, and valence. Here's an example of how expectancy feels: When you have a full-time job, you know that every 2 weeks you will be paid. This is what we call a high level of expectancy. You know you will be paid and the amount of time you have to wait for it to transpire. Another example is buying lottery tickets, and the expectation surrounding winning the big prize. You might be hopeful, but you certainly don't expect to win. Do you feel the difference between the two levels of expectancy?

When applied to sugar detox, expectancy is the belief that "I can do this. I can overcome my reliance on sugar".

Instrumentality is the belief that "If I do these things, I will have this result. When I limit sugar from my food, I will be proud of myself, create a better life for my children, and have a healthier body".

Valence, the next part of this theory, covers individual motivation. It can be something like this: "I want to detox from sugar because it is important to me to set a good example for my children and to feel better about myself" (Williams, n.d.).

These concepts are essential to help us understand why we have chosen detoxing from sugar as a valuable use of our energy and resources. Take some time to write down these 3 elements and how they apply to your life and motivation.

Summary: The theory of expectancy has 3 main pillars:

- expectancy (the belief that I can do it),

- instrumentality (I can see the end result of my effort),

- valence (personal motivation).

Theory of Goal-Setting and Motivation

In 1968, Edwin Locke published his groundbreaking "Goal Setting Theory of Motivation", commonly used today as a gold standard for goal-setting. His theory has been messaged in today's world to include an acronym to make it easier to remember: SMART (Tocino-Smith, 2021). Get your pen and paper out, because, as you know, it's crucial to write this stuff down.

S - Specific

Goals should be detailed, rather than general. For example, rather than say "I am becoming healthier, I am losing weight", you could say "I am limiting my sugar intake to only natural sugars. I am only purchasing and eating food that supports this goal". Then, you plan how to start this process immediately (you've already taken that step by reading this book!). Determine how your everyday life will change and how you will move toward achieving this goal. Also, make sure to write this down.

M - Measurable

This is how you determine whether you have achieved your goal(s), whether you are still in the process, or whether you need to redefine the steps you need to take (remember Confucius - the goal is always attainable, but perhaps the steps need to be more reasonable). This part of goal setting is *critical* to success - we need to start with small, easily attainable goals. Do not set your only goal as far as even a week down the road. Start with one day. "My goal for today is…" and choose one thing that will be a success for you toward detoxing from sugar. It could be "Today I remove all the chocolate from my home" (not by eating it all, ha-ha). Or "Today I choose to eat an apple, go for a walk, and start my evening routine". Ensure that within this goal-setting process, you also have small goals that will keep you motivated and create that feeling of accomplishment on an ongoing basis.

A - Acceptable

You must consider your goals acceptable insofar as they are in line with your values and that you identify with them. For example, you need to believe that eliminating your reliance on sugar won't affect your social life or your satisfaction with what you are eating, in the long run. You need to believe that your goal, and the things you need to do to achieve it, are "worth it".

R - Realistic

When we talk about whether something is realistic, this doesn't mean that it is easy or always comfortable. After all, nobody was ever proud of something that didn't require any effort. This is where we determine if your goals are something that you can achieve given your current circumstances and ability to commit time and energy to the goal and the steps. This loops back to the "Measurable" part of the goals, and why I am stressing how important it is to create small, achievable goals.

T- Timeframe

You must set dates, and write them down in your calendar. You need a concrete calendar to place your goals. Not ready to throw away all of your sugary foods today? That's ok. Decide when you can do that, and put it in your calendar. Prepare yourself for that day, and do it.

Finally, when you set your goals, use the present tense and use positive terms. Avoid words like "no," "not," "never." Instead, focus on what you *do* want to see, to happen, and to believe.

Summary: Consider the following for your goals:

• Specific (detailed),

• Measurable (to determine when the goal is achieved),

• Acceptable (fit into your lifestyle),

• Realistic (small, achievable),

• Timeframe (deadline with a specific date),

• Use the present tense to and use positive terms.

HAVE AN ATTITUDE OF GRATITUDE

Did you know that there is a huge correlation between being grateful and achieving health goals? Being thankful isn't just for Thanksgiving - it is something that we should be mindful of year-round and in everything we do. Being mindful of everything in our life is exactly as it should be (note that I didn't say "how we want it to be"). Here are some ways that being grateful supports us as we detox from sugar from a 2020 article called "Gratitude - A Mindset for Weight Loss" by C. Patrick:

- **Gratitude instills a sense of calm and makes us less reactive.**

When we feel stress, we often make poor choices about what we eat. We reach for what is easy, accessible, or what our past experiences make us believe will make us feel better. Being grateful can help calm our feelings of stress, therefore leaving the mental bandwidth to make better choices. When you feel overwhelmed, take the time to think about 3 things you are grateful for, and then decide IF you need to eat something, and if so, do you really need that sugary treat?

- **Gratitude helps us see our own worthiness.**

By creating a more positive outlook about ourselves and the world around us. Taking care of ourselves also means taking care of our bodies. When our eating is based on habit or driven by the idea that we aren't lovable, these emotions can sabotage our efforts to be healthier. Thinking about all of the incredible things our bodies can do and offer is a step toward loving ourselves, and it is natural to take care of those we love.

- **Gratitude improves our self-control.**

When we are grateful and mindful of the amazing things in our lives, this increases our ability to wait. Being able to "wait" is key to self-control, and therefore better decision-making about what we eat.

Similar to goal setting, a key component of gratitude is writing things down. Our brain processes and stores things better when we take the time to write them down.

Summary: There is a huge correlation between being grateful and achieving health goals. Be grateful for everything you have right now. Gratitude helps us:

- To be calm,

- To be positive,

- To improve self-control.

BE GENTLE WITH YOURSELF

Yes, we're moms, and we often feel like we can (and perhaps have to) "do it all". However, there is no pressure here other than what you are putting on yourself. You have already decided that you are worth a healthier lifestyle. The end result of your effort can be something like that: weight loss, consuming less processed foods, and setting a better example for your kids.

I am not asking you to be perfect. I'm not even expecting you to do it "my way", which is why this book is your guide and not your textbook. I am giving you grace and compassion as a busy mom in the hopes that you also give it to yourself.

Accept your realities and limitations. Remember we discussed realistic and achievable goals earlier in this Chapter? My goal for this book was to reach out to other moms who felt like the other sugar detox programs wouldn't work for them and give you a process that sees you and your busy life and shows you that I believe in you. When I use the word "limitations" as something to accept, I don't mean this word in a negative way. It simply refers to our realities as people who have other considerations beyond our desire to be healthier and to relinquish the hold that sugar has over us.

This is not an overnight fix. Something like that wouldn't work for me, and since you're reading this book, I think it's safe to say that it probably wouldn't work for you either. This is a journey where there may be times when you don't plan your day perfectly, and at that moment, you have a sugar-rich treat. This does not mean that you have failed. This means that you are human and imperfect, which is exactly what everyone else is. It means that you have been given the opportunity to look at how far you've come and all of the times that you did plan your day and did not end up eating that sugar-based food. And then the next time that happens, you'll realize that it's been even longer than the first time since it's happened.

And then, one day, you'll have the "ah-ha" moment when it occurs to you that you don't remember the last time you wanted sugar, where you felt like you needed it to get through the day. I want you to have that moment, and I believe that you will have it without a shadow of a doubt.

The knowledge you gain in this book and the steps outlined are your blueprint to success. But just like every blueprint, there are edits and ways to make it perfect for those who need it to work for them. Take what you've learned (and what I've learned) and make it work for your life. And absolutely expect to succeed.

Another way to be gentle with yourself is to surround yourself with those that support you. There will be skeptics and doubters, and those who simply don't understand why this is so important to you. This doesn't mean that they don't love or care for you. It simply means that, as I said, they don't understand. And that's ok. But do find those who have similar goals to you that can hold you up, cheer for you, and keep you accountable. I strongly encourage you to find additional support in our Facebook group "Weight loss for busy moms" (link to it you can find at the end of this book).

Summary: Accept your realities and limitations. All humans are imperfect. Love yourself as you are right now. Surround yourself with those that support you. *Join our Facebook group "Weight loss for busy moms" (link to it you can find at the end of this book).*

MOTIVATION

When we think about motivation, we're talking about your "why" and your reason for doing anything. Everything you do in your life has a "why" behind it, and the process of detoxing from sugar is no different. Until you know *exactly why* you are doing what you're doing, it's not something worth starting.

I believe our children and families can be part of our "why", but the main reason behind this process needs to be us. It needs to be <u>you</u>.

Perhaps you struggle with this idea, thinking that it is selfish. But do you remember when I mentioned pouring from an empty cup? How can you expect to pour your new lifestyle into your family if you haven't applied it to yourself first? If it's not important enough to do for you, then it won't stick when you try to do it for others. So start with yourself and be an example for your family.

Summary: Anything you do in life should have YOUR "why" behind it. Sugar detoxification is not different. Start with yourself, and later on, you will do it with the entire family.

Motivational Black Holes and Triggers

Because we are perfectly imperfect human beings, we do falter. However, as we have already learned, we must plan to succeed. For now, identify the situations or emotions where you are the most likely to crave sugar. For me, it was the mid-afternoon slump or late evenings where I felt like chocolate or other sweet snacks would give me the energy I needed to keep myself awake and get things done.

How did I overcome these moments? I had a plan. I identified the specific triggers for when I felt this need, and I had other foods on hand. My biggest challenge was sugar cravings at night when I needed to be awake. As a new mom, I had to replace my unhealthy sugary "emergency snacks" with healthier options like baby carrots. Usually, I had time to myself after everyone was in bed, and some of my projects would keep me up until 2:00 am. It was during these hours I struggled with my cravings. When my kids got older and slept through the night, I have changed my routine. Now I go to bed early (around 9:00 pm) and wake up at 4:30 am. I don't have cravings in the morning, and I can start my day eating a healthy, low GI meal. It worked for me, and you will figure out what works best for you!

For many others, I know the triggers can be emotional rather than situational. Emotional eating is not new or rare, so you are not alone in this. However, the way to overcome it is to identify what causes it and have a plan. If you know that, for example, talking to a certain person at work always causes you stress, have a plan for what you will do immediately after any conversation takes place. It's unlikely you're hungry at that moment, so your plan could be to go somewhere quiet and listen to a meditation on your phone. You could also spend time looking at photos of your loved ones. Or perhaps go for a walk outside or around the office, and take time to observe the little things that most overlook.

The things that trigger us to eat sugar are as varied as the stars in the sky, and you must identify your triggers. I'm asking you to get pen and paper again and write down every single event, emotion, time of day, or anything else that comes to mind as a reason to go to that drawer in your desk where you keep your sweet snacks.

For each one of these, come up with something from the SMART goals above (it doesn't have to be lengthy) that you will do differently. Every single one of these instances is a mini-goal and a small success toward the healthier you.

Summary: Take a paper and write down things that trigger you to eat sugar. It can be emotion, event, time of the day or anything else. Think about what else in this situation can replace sugar.

For example, if you think that eating sugar gives you energy, think about what else can provide you with energy. Probably, it will be a hot bath or just hugging your kid.

Each replacement will be one of the SMART goals that you will work on in the future.

LOFTY QUESTIONS

When we talk about success, goal-setting, and what we say to ourselves, there is a concept called "Lofty Questions" that provides us with a better method of achieving that success.

These are questions that you ask yourself and are positive, insightful, and encourage you to find a solution. So instead of saying "why do I always revert to sugar when I'm feeling sad?", you would ask yourself "why am I always worth the process of detoxing from sugar?" (Thomas, 2020).

So even if you're asking yourself a "why" question, the result is really a "how" answer. When you ask yourself a lofty question, your brain is forced to make a shift from a space of not knowing (and accepting this) to problem-solving. And our brains love to solve problems, so they get to work and dig up all of the reasons why and then help us figure out the how. These questions provide you with the roadmap for your current situation and new and exciting destinations (Thomas, 2020).

When it comes to lofty questions, 4 key elements must be in place (Thomas, 2020):

1. The question must be phrased positively.

The example above is just one you can refer to, but another could be "why will I always be successful at detoxing from sugar?" rather than "why will this be so difficult for me?".

2. It must be a question.

This is how you get your brain to start working to solve or confirm what you've said, because it's not a statement or a fact.

3. Include the words "always" or "at all times".

This plants the seed of certainty in your mind, where your mind hears that your success isn't an option and it isn't dependent on time or circumstance.

4. Be in a relaxed, meditative state.

For these questions to be truly effective, you need to remove distractions and be committed to the answers that your brain will come up with

---

Summary: The concept of "Lofty Questions" provides us with a better method of achieving success. When we say a positive statement (also known as affirmation), it might trigger doubts in our brain. In contrast, when you ask yourself a lofty question, your brain is forced to make a shift to problem-solving.

We have covered several elements of preparing your mind for success in our path of detoxing from sugar. Each of these revolves around you and your belief in your worthiness to succeed. If you are ever in doubt about who believes in you, take a look at this book, because I do. And because you took the step of reading this book… YOU DO.

Now it is time to move to meal planning, where we will discuss how to plan your entire day and have less sugar cravings.

3

STEP 3 - PLAN AND ENJOY YOUR MEALS

Our primary goal with a low-sugar lifestyle is to regulate our blood. Once we have detoxed from our reliance on sugar, this will come much more easily and naturally. We go through the actual detox process in the next Chapter, so let's focus on how our meals should look during our day.

Our new low-sugar lifestyle will support our health. As we go through our well-planned day, it's essential to focus on having food on hand that keeps our metabolism from crashing because we're overly hungry. Planning our meals and snacks based on the GI/GL chart is a good place to start.

It'll happen - you will have that moment where you think you need sugar to get through a tough spot.

The keys to managing these cravings are:

- have food on hand that will healthily satisfy the craving,
- have a plan of your meals and snacks ahead of time,
- focus on enjoying the food and company.

And we will cover them in this Chapter.

IMPORTANT HIGHLIGHTS ABOUT FOOD

You're educated and prepared, and now we're ready to talk about the food that will be part of your new lifestyle. We'll keep it simple, and what's outlined in this Chapter will be realistic and supportive. It is the beginning of your success!

Where to Find Healthy Food Choices (Shop "Outside of the Store")

As you know, the food industry spends a *lot* of money on marketing and perfecting the psychology behind what you purchase and why. They are attempting to make your decisions for you, essentially by making you believe what they're telling you. But who is going to decide what you eat from this day forward? The prepared, newly educated, determined YOU.

Perhaps you've noticed this before, perhaps not: natural, unprocessed food is always on the outside border of the grocery stores. Don't tell the grocery stores that we've figured this out - they'll start mixing things up to get us to buy the processed stuff with big marketing budgets!

You still may need things from the inside aisles. But try to stick to the "outside of the store" as much as possible. This is where you'll find your produce, grains, lean proteins, and dairy products. This is where you'll find the low GI/GL foods. Oh, and the flowers are often on the outside too. Buy yourself some flowers while you're touring the outside of the grocery store - because you deserve it!

Venturing into the inside aisles, as I mentioned, isn't terrible. But this is where you find the sugary beverages, the sugar-laden cereals, and other processed and frozen foods. (Disclaimer - just because a food is frozen does not make it "bad". Frozen veggies and fruits can have a lot of excellent and healthy uses).

Summary: Be smarter than food manufactures, do not fall on their tricks. When you do your grocery, stick to the outside of the store as much as possible. This is where you'll find fruits and vegetables, grains, lean proteins, and dairy products.

Fat-Burning Food (Buy This Stuff)

There is no quick fix to burn all of the calories you've eaten that day. But some food and beverages can support your goals toward detoxing from sugar, and when eaten in combination with low GI/GL food, they will nourish your body and help you achieve (and maintain) success!

So, which food can we add to our lifestyle instead of sugary ones? For now, let's cover "fat-burning food". It sounds great, especially if you are aiming to lose weight as well. But in reality, you should not expect too much fat burning by eating such food. The term "fat-burning food" is not entirely accurate. No food will burn fat. Our body burns fat when we need energy for essential processes like breathing, digestion, pumping blood, etc. It is important to understand that this food temporarily boosts your metabolism and slightly increases fat burning by our body. The results depend on your age, current weight, and lifestyle. (Spritzler, 2021a).

To provide a bit more insight on this food, let's break it down and discuss some specific food and their benefits:

Apple cider vinegar

Apple cider vinegar contains acetic acid. That acid promotes fat burning. Researches are limited, but 2 studies suggest consuming it for losing a small amount of body fat. Limiting your dose to 2 tablespoons per day is important to avoid digestive distress. (Spritzler, 2021a).

Celery

Probably you heard about the "negative calories theory". The idea of this theory is that some high-fibre vegetables require more calories to digest than they contain. But studies on this subject are limited, and those that exist do not confirm it. Here is research from 2014. 15 women eat 100 grams of celery (this is about 16 calories), and within the next 3 hours, they burn around 14 calories digesting it. So, most consumed calories were burned, but they did not get negative. However, such high-fibre vegetables create a calory deficit, leading to fat burning (Spritzler, 2021a).

Coconut oil

Research shows that coconut oil is less likely to be stored as fat in comparison with animal and other plant-based fats. The strongest boost of metabolism lasts the first two weeks after you start to consume it. Lean people have a greater metabolic rate than overweight. Because coconut oil has a lot of calories, over time, it can contribute to weight gain. So, if you decide to experiment with coconut oil, switch to other fats with time. Be aware of possible side effects like gas or diarrhea (Spritzler, 2021a).

Coffee/Non-herbal tea

Each of these is a great source of caffeine. And caffeine is known as an energy booster. Together with energy, it can increase metabolism. Study shows that people who drink 100 – 200 ml of caffeine (approximately 2 cups) have increased metabolic rate by 3 – 7% for several hours. And if intake was increased to 600 ml for 12 hours, then calorie-burning was increased by 8 – 11%. But please, be careful with that. 600 ml of caffeine is a significant number, and you can have side effects like insomnia. In addition, this amount is not acceptable for people with heart conditions. And remember that we are aiming for a low sugar lifestyle, so the amount of sugar you add to those beverages should be limited (Spritzler, 2021a).

Eggs

Eggs are other pure-protein food. There was some controversy surrounding the high cholesterol in eggs, but studies have proven that there is no evidence to support that eating cholesterol causes high cholesterol.

According to the journal Nutrition Research, eating eggs early in the day has a beneficial effect on how hungry we get and our food choices as we go through our day (Kandola, 2019a).

Fatty/Oily fish

Sardines, salmon, herring, and other oily (fatty) fish contain omega-3 fatty acids. This is why they're called "fatty fish" - because of their high levels of healthy fatty acids, not because they have a lot of fat! In addition, fish is high in protein. Both omega-3 and protein are linked to losing body fat (Kandola, 2019a).

Ginger

Ginger is a spice that can help you to burn slightly more calories. There is no harm in consuming ginger, and little effect on weight loss. A review found that ginger contributes to losing abdominal fat. (Spritzler, 2021a).

Green tea/Green tea extract

Those beverages contain approximately 20 – 40 ml of caffeine per cup. In addition, they have antioxidants that also contribute to a slight increase in metabolic rate. However, no studies confirm that just consuming green tea/extract will increase fat/calorie burning. Only combination with resistance training gives better results; on average, burning an additional 260 calories per day (Spritzler, 2021a). Walking, running, and squats are some examples of resistance training.

Hot peppers

If you like spicy peppers: cayenne, chilli, and jalapeno, you can take advantage of it. One study found that by adding those to your food, you can expect to burn additional 70 calories per day. And in contrast to caffeine, which works better for lean people, hot peppers give better results for heavier people (Spritzler, 2021a).

Nuts

Nuts are high in fat and calories. Because of this, many assume that they should be avoided if you're trying to eat healthier. However, nuts are perfect for adding to our daily food for a low-sugar lifestyle. Both protein and good fats are great for controlling hunger over long periods, making us less likely to reach for a sugary snack (Kandola, 2019b).

Nuts are great options for a low-sugar menu. They contain high levels of healthy unsaturated fats that perform important bodily functions, such as supporting cell growth and protecting organs, like the heart. Nuts are also rich in protein, which we know builds muscle and leaves us feeling fuller longer. To ensure that we limit excess calorie intake, consider one serving of nuts to be a handful or about a ¼ cup (Kandola, 2019b).

In the January 2019 Medical News Today Newsletter, Aaron Kandola outlines the 5 best nuts to support a low-sugar diet. Keep in mind that these are raw or plain roasted, without added salt or sugars. They are (Kandola, 2019b):

- Almonds
- Walnuts
- Cashews
- Pistachios
- Peanuts

Yogurt

Plain Greek yogurt is an excellent for our low-sugar lifestyle. The Nutrition Journal published a study from 2014 that shows eating high-protein yogurt can benefit us by controlling appetite, lowering hunger, and we might eat less food entirely (Kandola, 2019a).

Summary: Even though "fat-burning" food sounds good, it is inaccurate. First of all, it is our body, not food is burning fat. Second, some food can temporarily increase metabolic rate and contribute to burning extra calories (fat). This food includes apple cider vinegar, celery, coconut oil, coffee/non-herbal tea, eggs, fatty/oily fish, ginger, green tea/green tea extract, hot peppers, nuts, and yogurt.

Do not expect too much weight loss with such food, be aware of the side effects of some food. It is just an idea about what you can consider including in your diet instead of sugary food.

Filling Food

Some food, called "high-satisfaction food", help us feel fuller (satiated) and more satisfied, which helps control our appetite and regulate our blood sugars. (Live Naturally Magazine, 2013). While we search for delicious, low-sugar, nutritious foods, let's focus on high-satisfaction food that tends to fill us up but is low on the GI/GL charts. The great news is that filling food tends to score lower on the GI! And this food is excellent for the time when we typically reach for sugary food as our "quick fix".

Apples

Research has shown that when healthy adults ate one medium-sized apple about 15 minutes before their meal, they ate an average of 15% less calories during the meal. Apples contain a good amount of soluble fibre and nutrients (Live Naturally Magazine, 2013). Low on the GI, apples are a convenient, portable, and delicious snack or addition to meals that will make you feel fuller!

Beans and legumes

Beans, especially chickpeas, lentils, soybeans, black beans, and pinto beans, are great plant-based satisfying food. They're convenient because the canned variety is equally as healthy as dried. They can be added to salads, rice, whole-grain pasta, and spreads (Live Naturally Magazine, 2013).

Fish

The omega-3 healthy fats and protein combined create an even higher level of satiety (Live Naturally Magazine, 2013). Fish is your best protein option.

Green veggies

Leafy vegetables like spinach, kale, lettuces, and others provide us with vitamins, protein, and fibre. Live Naturally Magazine suggests having at least 5 servings of vegetables per day and 2 of them with leafy greens (Live Naturally Magazine, 2013).

Nuts and seeds

Almonds, cashews, walnuts, sunflower and pumpkin seeds are other great source of protein. They are all handy for snacks, salads, soups or your morning oatmeal or yogurt (Live Naturally Magazine, 2013).

Sweet potatoes

According to Live Naturally Magazine, sweet potatoes are great filling food and can help stabilize blood sugar (Live Naturally Magazine, 2013). And this is our main goal for a low-sugar lifestyle. Just remember to keep your portion size not more than 80 grams.

Whole grains

Oatmeal, oat bran, wheat pasta, and wheat bran can increase feelings of fullness until our next meal. Once again, do not forget about portion size (Live Naturally Magazine, 2013). Recommended portion size is around 50 grams.

Summary: Just because we are eating lower-sugar and lower-calorie food doesn't mean that we need to feel hungry all the time. The filling food mentioned above will support us as we journey toward removing our reliance on sugar by keeping us fuller, and giving us the satisfaction we need when we eat.

Great Food for a Low-Sugar Lifestyle

As you already know, our primary goal for a low-sugar lifestyle is maintaining a low sugar intake. And if at this point, you are overloaded with information and terminology that we have covered so far, then I suggest getting back to basics. A low-sugar lifestyle usually means eating what nature gives to us and eliminating processed food containing added sugar.

Summary: Do not let information overwhelm you. Gradually remove processed food from your menu and enjoy the fresh produce that nature gives us.

Smart Food Swaps

In Appendix 3, you can find food "swaps" that can be used in our low-sugar lifestyle.

These swaps consider GI/GL and the amount of sugar in the foods listed. One of the best ways to start and continue our lower-sugar lifestyle is to find ways to satisfy our brains and taste buds, while still staying true to our goals. We can continue to eat things that provide what our addicted brains are looking for, while almost "tricking" them into believing we're eating sugar!

Summary: Start using food "swaps" as you go towards your new lifestyle.

Water

It's perhaps not a surprise that you need to drink water for a healthy lifestyle. This is no exception to detoxing from sugar and our new low-sugar lifestyle.

A generic recommendation is to drink 8 glasses of water a day.

It's easy to remember, and a reasonable goal (Mayo Clinic, 2018).

More specific minimum daily intake of water:
(Mayo Clinic, 2020b):
Women — 11.5 cups, or 92 ounces, or 2.7 litres
Men — 15.5 cups, or 124 ounces, or 3.7 litres

This varies based on activity level, environment (dry or humid climate), overall health, pregnancy and breast-feeding (Mayo Clinic, 2020b). There is currently no agreement on how much water children should drink because so many factors impact these numbers.

If you like a calculation <u>beyond general suggestions</u>:
Daily water intake (in ounces) = Your weight (in pounds) / 2
Daily water intake (in cups) = Daily water intake (in ounces) / 8

If we use this formula, a 130-pound person should drink 8 cups (glasses) of water.

130 / 2 = 65 ounces

65 / 8 ounces (1 cup) = 8 cups (Neal, 2020).

Water makes up 50% to 70% of your body weight, and your body needs water to survive because every cell, tissue, and organ in your body needs it to function. Lack of water can cause dehydration, causing your body to be unable to carry out its normal functions (Mayo Clinic, 2020b).

Summary: Pick any method mentioned above to calculate your daily water intake. And make your goal to stick to it as close as possible.

Tips and Tricks for Drinking Enough Water

There are many ways to remember to drink more water, even when we're busy or on the road, running from one activity to another. As far as your vehicle is concerned, keep a bottle of water at all times, and have it in your cupholder. When it starts to get low, take it inside, fill it up, and put it in front of your door, so you don't forget to replace it. Drinking water while you're driving is one of the easiest ways to keep your hydration up!

Mayo Clinic's 2018 "Tips for Drinking More Water" gives some other ways to help you drink enough water:

- **Flavour it**

Add fruit to your water. Lemons, limes, oranges, cucumber, watermelon, strawberries, and herbs are delicious ways to add flavour.

• Tie it into a routine and create a new habit

Drink a glass of water every time you brush your teeth, eat, or drive your car. Find something that makes sense for you!

• Challenge a friend or family member

Kick off a healthy competition with a friend, your spouse, kids. And see who can meet their water goal most often.

• Alternate your drinks

If you can't give up soda or juice completely just yet, try alternating it with water. Each time you want a glass of soda or juice, start from water and then switch to another drink.

Summary: In your daily life, start drinking water to meet recommendations. Find the ways that keep you on track. Flavour water, creating a routine, competing with family members, and alternating drinks are just a few examples that you can use in your journey.

Make Water Your Drink of Choice

Beyond the physiological reasons above to drink water, I'm going to outline just how much sugar there is in other types of beverages and why water should always be your main drink of choice. Here's an idea of how much sugar is in soda pop and other sugary drinks (a 12oz serving - one regular sized can) from Harvard's School of Public Health 2012 article "How Sweet Is It?":

- Coca-Cola Classic (41 grams = 10 teaspoons)
- Fanta Orange (45 grams = 13 teaspoons)
- Pepsi Cola (41 grams = 10 teaspoons)
- Schweppes Tonic Water (35 grams = 8 teaspoons)
- Low Sodium V8 100% Vegetable Juice (12 grams = 3 teaspoons)
- Minute Maid Orange Juice (41 grams = 10 teaspoons)

- Mott's Plus for Kids' Health Juice Apple Grape (48 grams = 11 teaspoons)
- POM Wonderful 100% Pomegranate Juice (60 grams = 14 teaspoons)
- Minute Maid Lemonade (42 grams = 10 teaspoons)
- Red Bull (40 grams = 10 teaspoons)
- Lipton Brisk Green Tea (34 grams = 8 teaspoons)
- Nestea Sweetened Lemon Iced Tea (35 grams = 8 teaspoons)
- Nesquik Ready-to-Drink Chocolate Milk, Reduced Fat (48 grams = 11 teaspoons)
- Silk Chocolate Soymilk (32 grams = 8 teaspoons)

Beyond the very high sugar amount in these beverages, the calories are considered "empty calories, " meaning zero nutritional value. This needs to be differentiated from the previously discussed foods that burn fat. Although our bodies do need to do the work to break down the calories in sugary beverages, the high amount of sugar in them means that literally, the only thing we are getting from them is pure added sugar.

Remember that juices like apple juice don't have a place in our new low-sugar lifestyle as well. Start gradually removing them from your menu.

Summary: Giving up on soft drinks and juices can be one of your main goals. Because this type of drink has "empty calories" and gives us a significant amount of pure added sugar.

MEAL PLANNING IS PLANNING TO SUCCEED

Having a plan is essential - it is the foundation on which success is built. Your plan outlines objectives and solidifies what you want to achieve both on paper and in your mind. You already know how to create a plan from the previous Chapter (in the section about goal setting). Let's apply the general principles from that section to meal planning.

We will cover a template for your plate with general portion sizes to stick to. Our focus will be on filling your plate with lean proteins, fibre-rich vegetables, grains/starches, and naturally sweet fruits that will leave you feeling satisfied.

Next, I will cover some examples of food that can be considered part of our "plate template", simple meal ideas, and how often we should be eating or "meal frequency".

A Template for your Plate

There are many plate templates that you can find on the Internet. The one provided below considers Diabetes Food Hub and U.S. Department of Agriculture and U.S. Department of Health and Human Services recommendations and combines the best of both. The plate template below emphasizes on sugar levels and GI/GL. This consideration is crucial in our low-sugar lifestyle because we are not simply looking to eat "healthier" things. We also want to consume things that are low in sugar.

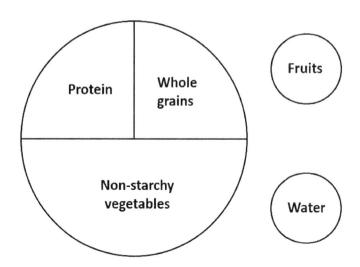

Figure 2. 9-inch plate template (Diabetes Food Hub, 2020; U.S. Department of Agriculture and U.S. Department of Health and Human Services, 2020)

When we talk about portion sizes and what your meals should look like, use these proportions to help make healthy and low-sugar meals or snacks.

- Half of the plate is non-starchy vegetables: include low GI/GL choices.
- One-quarter of the plate is whole grains (whole grains have a lower GI than grains).
- One-quarter of the plate is protein.
- Fruits are out of the plate because we are focused on a low-sugar lifestyle. However, in moderation, low GI/GL fruits are acceptable. It is preferable to consume more vegetables as a part of each meal or snack. In addition, fruits can be excluded from some meals of the day.
- Water is out of the plate because it is recommended to drink water more often than you eat. And we already covered how much you should drink.

Here are a few important notes about the plate template:

- Recommended plate size is 9-inch. So, it is good to have such a plate at home to visually see recommended portion sizes (Diabetes Food Hub, 2020).

- How to deal with combination dishes like a casserole, sandwich, soup, etc.? You can still apply the plate method while preparing food for your meal. You need to identify food groups and imagine where they fit into the plate in the correct proportions (Diabetes Food Hub, 2020).
- Fruits are optional, and you can choose to skip them with some meals or have them on the side with the main meal.
- If you need snacks between meals, keep in mind that the plate template applies for the entire day. So, it is totally fine to have one snack just protein and another just fruit. The main idea is that all snacks for the day will fit into the plate template in the correct proportions.

Summary: Here is a generic plate template:

- Half of the plate is non-starchy vegetables.

- One-quarter of the plate is whole grains.

- One-quarter of the plate is protein.

- Fruits are out of the plate but allowed low GI/GL fruits in moderation.

- Water is out of the plate because it is recommended to drink more often than eat.

And few things to remember:

- Consider the same proportion for combination dishes like soup.
- The plate template for snacks is for the entire day.

What's on My Plate?

Below are some examples of each type of food that are present on the plate template. Remember to choose low GI/GL food.

Non-starchy vegetables (Diabetes Food Hub, 2020)

- Asparagus
- Brussels sprouts
- Broccoli
- Cabbage (green, red, bok choy, Chinese)
- Carrots
- Cauliflower
- Celery
- Cucumber
- Eggplant
- Green beans
- Leafy greens (basil, collards, dill, kale, mint, mustard greens, parsley)
- Mushrooms
- Okra
- Peapods, snow peas, and sugar snap peas
- Peppers (bell peppers, hot peppers)
- Salad greens (lettuce, arugula, other salad mixes)
- Spinach
- Squash (yellow, spaghetti, zucchini)
- Tomato

The majority of non-starchy vegetables do not have a GI rating. This is because they have a very low amount of carbohydrates. It is safe to consume them in our low-sugar lifestyle. Carrot usually has a low GI, but cooking it (and the longer you cook it) significantly increases GI.

Whole grains

Let's explain the meaning of "whole" grains. A grain is a seed from a plant. Each seed has outer layers: bran, germ, and endosperm. These layers contain vitamins, minerals, fibre, carbohydrates, protein, and healthy unsaturated fats. "Whole" grains have those layers; that is why it is our best choice. These layers are removed from the processed or refined grains, so the nutrition value becomes lower. For example, the milling process mechanically removes bran and germ, and together with them, we lose vitamin B, E, minerals, fatty acids, and fibre (Cleveland Clinic, 2020b).

Here are some shopping tips for buying "whole" grains (Cleveland Clinic, 2020b):

- Read the list of ingredients on the label and give a preference to products with the first listed ingredient "whole grain".
- Avoid products with the phrase "enriched" or "refined."
- Search for the "Whole Grain" stamp from the nonprofit Whole Grains Council. This will

guarantee that food contains at least a half serving of "whole grains".

And now, we will move to the most common list of "whole" grains (Cleveland Clinic, 2020b):

- 100% whole-wheat bread
- 100% whole-grain (wheat, corn, oat) cereals
- 100% whole-wheat flatbread
- 100% whole-wheat tortillas
- Barley
- Bulgur
- Brown rice
- Chia seeds
- Kasha
- Oatmeal (steel cut, instant or old fashioned)
- Quinoa
- Whole-wheat couscous
- Whole-wheat pasta
- Whole-wheat pastry flour
- Wild rice

Protein

Protein food can be divided into two main groups (Diabetes Food Hub, 2020):

- Animal sources,
- Plant-based sources

As a reminder, **cheese, eggs, fish, meat, and poultry do not have Glycemic Index (GI)** because of a very small amount of carbohydrates in this food. It is the perfect choice for a low-sugar lifestyle (Foster-Powell et al., 2002).

Examples of animal sources of protein include (Diabetes Food Hub, 2020):

- Beef
- Cheese
- Chicken
- Cottage cheese
- Fish (cod, salmon, tilapia, tuna)
- Deli meats
- Eggs
- Pork
- Shellfish (clams, lobster, mussels, scallops, shrimp)
- Turkey

Plant-based sources of protein (Diabetes Food Hub, 2020):

- Beans
- Edamame
- Falafel
- Hummus
- Lentils
- Nuts
- Nut butter
- Plant-based meat substitutes
- Tofu

Fruits

Fruits are out of the plate template because we aim low-sugar lifestyle. However, fresh fruits are a much better choice than sweets from processed sugar. We already stressed that fresh fruits in moderation are acceptable for our goals in this book. And "moderation" for us means that we consume low GI/GL fruits, and we respect serving size.

We already learned that:

- Values of GI/GL can vary in different sources (in this book, we will stick to values from Appendix 2),

- Some fruits like **lime and lemon do not have GI,**
- Fruits like watermelon and pineapple have a high GI, but if we consider serving size (120 grams), GL becomes low, and it fits a low-sugar lifestyle.

The main resource that I used for Appendix 2 did not contain information about GI/GL for raspberry and blueberry. But in my family, those are my favourite, and kids love them. So, it was worth doing further research and finding out those numbers. And here we go (Mad About Berries, 2020):

- Blueberries: GI = 53; Serving size = 150 g; GL = 9.6,
- Raspberries: GI = 32; Serving size = 150 g; GL = 2.6

Based on the information above, let's provide a list of fresh fruits suitable for our goals. If the fruit has a moderate or high Glycemic Index, we provide a serving size that puts the same fruit into low Glycemic Load, which means that we can include it on the menu, but we should respect that portion size.

- Apple
- Apricot (120 g)
- Banana (green)
- Blueberries (150 g)
- Cantaloupe (120 g)
- Grapefruit
- Lemon
- Lime
- Mango (120 g)
- Orange
- Peach (120 g)
- Pear
- Plum
- Raspberries (150 g)

Summary: Use examples of the food from our 9-inch plate template as inspiration. Explore and experiment in your kitchen but keep in mind your goals. I believe YOU can improve your current diet!

Meal Ideas

Looking back at our plate template and considering the food listed above, we can be creative and include many different healthy, satisfying, and low GI/GL food in our low-sugar lifestyle. Remember that this is not a cook-book, and I want to provide just general principles and templates witch you can apply to your family. And of course, use common sense. For example, we all know that kids need less food, so a 9-inch plate template needs modification. As a mom, you also know that toddlers prefer to have their food separated and only with time they will start eating salads, soups, etc. And now, I would like to give you a few of my favourite meal ideas to show you how you can convert a plate template into a real meal.

Breakfast

- Eggs scrambled with cheese and tomatoes, wrapped in a whole-grain tortilla, served with apple slices. (**Protein**: eggs, cheese; **whole grains**: tortilla; **non-starchy vegetables**: tomatoes; **fruits**: apple)

- Smoothie from Greek yogurt, raspberry, and cauliflower (blanched/frozen cauliflower is an excellent option to add a creamy texture, and you don't taste it!) with a piece of dry snack bread. (**Protein**: yogurt; **whole grains**: dry snack bread; **non-starchy vegetables**: cauliflower; **fruits**: raspberry)

- Overnight oats with yogurt and blueberry, with some radishes or cucumbers on the side. (**Protein**: yogurt; **whole grains**: oats; **non-starchy vegetables**: cucumber, radish; **fruits**: blueberry)

- Baked egg frittata with bulgur, tomatoes, zucchini, and spinach, topped with cheese and sliced orange on the side (**Protein**: eggs, cheese; **whole grains**: bulgur; **non-starchy vegetables**: tomatoes, zucchini, spinach; **fruits**: orange)

- Kefir with chia seeds and frozen raspberry, with a baby carrot on the side. (**Protein**: kefir; **whole grains**: chia seeds; **non-starchy vegetables**: baby carrot; **fruits**: frozen raspberry)

Lunch

- Charcuterie: lean meats, cheeses, chopped multicolour peppers, cucumbers, nuts, crackers, sliced pears, and apples. (**Protein**: meats, cheeses, nuts; **whole grains**: crackers; **non-starchy vegetables**: peppers, cucumbers; **fruits**: apples, pears)

- Salad with leafy greens, beans, dry bread, and a home-made dressing made from blended cottage cheese, sour cream, and fresh herbs. (**Protein**: beans, cottage cheese, sour cream, **whole grains**: dry bread; **non-starchy vegetables**: leafy greens; **fruits**: none)

- Sandwich with sourdough/spelt bread, lean meat, raw veggies: lattice, cucumber and a home-made dressing made from Greek yogurt and dill. (**Protein**: lean meat, Greek yogurt; **whole grains**: sourdough/spelt bread; **non-starchy vegetables**: lattice, dill, cucumber; **fruits**: none)

- Tabbouleh salad (chopped parsley, mint, green onion, tomatoes; bulgur; home-made dressing from olive oil and freshly squeezed lemon) with a boiled egg on the side (**Protein**: egg; **whole grains**: bulgur; **non-starchy vegetables**: parsley, mint, green onion, tomatoes; **fruits**: lemon)

Dinner

- Grilled salmon and eggplant with freshly squeezed lemon, with a side of brown rice, and sliced fresh peaches (**Protein**: salmon; **whole grains**: brown rice; **non-starchy vegetables**: eggplant; **fruits**: peach)

- Whole-wheat couscous with spinach salad, grilled chicken, and fresh strawberries. (**Protein**: chicken; **whole grains**: couscous; **non-starchy vegetables**: spinach; **fruits**: strawberries)

- Whole-wheat pasta with homemade meat and vegetable sauce with a side of blueberries. (**Protein**: ground beef (in the sauce); **whole grains**: whole-wheat pasta; **non-starchy vegetables**: tomatoes, carrot, pepper (in the sauce); **fruits**: blueberries)

- Bell pepper stuffed with ground beef and pork, brown rice, chopped tomatoes, basil, and all spices. (**Protein**: ground beef and pork; **whole grains**: brown rice; **non-starchy vegetables**: tomatoes, basil; **fruits**: none)

Snacks

- Baby carrot (**non-starchy vegetable**)
- Cauliflower with a dip from sour cream and dill (**Protein**: sour cream; **non-starchy vegetable**: cauliflower, dill)
- Cottage cheese (**protein**)
- Cherry tomatoes (**non-starchy vegetables**)
- Cucumber with a dip from Greek yogurt and dill (**Protein**: Greek yogurt; **non-starchy vegetable**: cucumber, dill)
- Fresh fruits with low GI (see list above) (**fruits**)
- Home-made oat bar with nuts and berries (**Protein**: nuts; **whole grains**: oats; **fruits**: berries)
- Nuts (**protein**)
- Pita with hummus (**Protein**: hummus; **whole grains**: pita)
- Popcorn (lightly seasoned, air-popped) (**whole grains**)
- Slice of cheese (**protein**)
- Sliced apple with nut butter (**Protein**: nut butter; **fruits**: apple)
- Plain yogurt (**protein**)

Remember that snacks should respect plate template not individually but for an entire day.

Summary: Above, you can find a few examples of meal ideas for breakfast, lunch, dinner, and snacks that respect the plate template.

Meal Frequency

From my own experience, if I eat less than three times a day, I overeat or choose high-sugar food. A study supports a regular meal pattern. But eating breakfast followed by multiple smaller daily meals better control blood sugar levels than eating fewer, larger meals (Ahola et al, 2019).

Because we are used to eating sugary and possibly processed food, it may take some time to get used to nature's wonderful natural sweetness. The food we are "supposed" to be eating might taste a bit dull, but your tastebuds will adapt quickly, and you will love your new sources of sweetness!

Summary: Eating 3 times a day can help keep you full and reduce hunger and cravings.

Start the Day Right – Breakfast

We have learned about what our bodies require and how sugar actually can work against us. Another important foundation is how we start each day - and what we eat for breakfast.

Eating breakfast is what gets our bodies going, and gets our metabolism started for the day. You may be aware that the word "breakfast" comes from "breaking the fast" - and our metabolism almost shuts down while we are resting and "fasting" overnight. We already covered the best food to eat that takes our bodies the most energy to burn, so we need to focus on this food first thing in the morning (and for every meal!). Breakfast restores and replenishes the energy stores and nutrients in your body (Cleveland Clinic, 2020a).

Many of you might not love the idea of eating in the morning, and the thought of digging into a hearty breakfast might completely turn you off, so I'll cover some easy breakfasts that won't feel like they're a lot of work and won't make you turn up your nose. Also, as busy moms, we are often so focused on getting our families to eat something in the morning that we might forget about ourselves. We suddenly realize it's almost noon, and we're famished. This is where we risk making poor decisions because we're already hungry, and we want to avoid an overwhelming feeling of hunger. I mentioned eating every 3-4 hours, and one of the purposes of this is to prevent feeling overly hungry and making poor choices. When our bodies create the "hunger signal", this means that we are entering into a fasting phase, and our metabolism is starting to slow down (Cleveland Clinic, 2020a). Making good food choices right from the start of the day keeps our metabolisms high!

Back to breakfast - most people who skip breakfast aren't doing so because they aren't hungry. It's because they're rushed for time. Remember how we talked about insulin and how it responds to sugar? Mornings are when your body is the most insulin sensitive, meaning that it uses blood sugar more effectively. Because of this, it's the perfect opportunity to choose grains and starches that are high in fibre, like dense bread and bran-based cereals. If you're one who usually skips breakfast or eats something that doesn't properly fuel your body, what is stopping you from eating a healthy breakfast? Preparing your food or kitchen in advance takes very little time and removes the morning stress of figuring out what to eat (Cleveland Clinic, 2020a). It could be as simple as putting the toaster on the counter with the bread, a plate, and your toppings right beside it. Another great way to make breakfast easy and healthy is to make overnight oats. You can find many delicious low GI recipes online. Just be aware of the fruits you're putting in and make sure they are as low as possible on the GI/GL charts.

Summary: Eating breakfast gets our metabolism started for the day. Our body is most insulin sensitive in the morning, so our body uses blood sugar more effectively. Prepare food for breakfast in advance to avoid the "morning rush".

Don't Forget the "Little Things": Snacks for the Rest of the Day

We already covered some strategies on how to choose food for our more substantial meals:

- Keep processed sugar under recommended quantity,
- Give preference to food with low GI/GL,
- Include "fat-burning" food and filling food,
- The plate template gives you an idea about the ratio of different types of food that you are consuming.

It's not unrealistic to say that cravings typically show up between meals. I believe most of us don't sit down to an entire meal of sugary foods. Our high sugar intake is more based on what we eat or drink to get us through the day. When we've hit a slump or a craving, it's typically in the form of a snack.

Eating filling, high-fibre, high protein, low GI/GL food is the best way to combat cravings and unhealthy snacking. We have already covered each type of this food. But I have a few more things to say about protein.

After eating, our metabolism rate (calorie burning) increases because our body needs to digest food. Research shows that increase is about 20-30% to digest protein, 5-10% to digest carbs, 3% to digest fat. When you consume 100 grams of protein (400 calories), your body will burn 80-120 calories to digest it. The study confirms that eating protein can help you to burn body fat (Spritzler, 2021b).

So, if you give preference to protein during the day instead of sugary food, you will feel full and satisfied for longer. Plus, you will have a bonus: you will help your body burn fat. You already know examples of protein food. But not all proteins are equal.

In the article "The best high-protein foods for weight loss" by Franziska Spritzler, I found interesting information about protein as a percentage of calories for different food. A bigger number means that food provides more protein per calorie (Spritzler, 2021b).

Here are some numbers from this article (Spritzler, 2021b):

- White fish - 82
- Plain nonfat (0%) Greek yogurt - 77
- Top sirloin steak - 69
- Chicken breast with skin - 63
- Spinach - 57
- Extra-firm tofu - 48
- Lentils - 42
- Brussels sprouts - 38
- Lamb chops - 36
- Eggs - 34
- Chickpeas - 26
- Cheddar - 24
- Almonds - 15

The more you adapt the ideas mentioned above, the less carving you will have during the day. But it takes time to get there. Meanwhile, consider the following protein snacks during the day (Calihan, 2021):

- Almonds and almond butter
- Canned fish and seafood
- Cheese
- Chia pudding
- Cottage cheese (1% milkfat)

- Eggs
- Greek yogurt (plain, 2% milkfat)
- Ground beef – sliders and meatballs
- Lupini beans
- Parmesan crisps
- Peanuts and peanut butter
- Pumpkin seeds
- Soybeans (black)
- Tofu
- Zero-sugar jerky

Prepare snacks ahead of time. Have healthy snacks in your vehicle at all times. These could be nuts or beef jerky, both high in protein and low on the GI/GL charts. Be careful of premade trail mixes because they often contain sugar-coated ingredients. Also, while low-GI/GL fruit is fine to eat in moderation, dried fruits can push us over our added sugar needs because it is much easier to eat a lot of dried fruit than fresh fruit.

Summary: Usually, we feel cravings between meals. Eating filling, high-fibre, high protein, low GI/GL food is the best way to combat cravings and unhealthy snacking.

Finishing the Day

If you find that you're hungry or craving sugary snacks at the end of the day, we have covered many healthy and low-sugar options that won't uproot your success for that day. To reinforce the importance of planning, we need to have this food on-hand and easily accessible, so we aren't tempted to reach our old crutch - sugar!

Every person is different, and the body will respond differently. According to Fletcher's 2020 article that delves into how our blood sugar levels change throughout the night, it is due mainly to two processes (Fletcher, 2020):

• The Dawn phenomenon

Between the hours of (roughly) 3:00 am and 8:00 am, our blood sugar levels rise as part of the process of waking up. This can cause high blood sugar levels in the morning, making our first meal of the day exceptionally important.

- **The Somogyi effect**

Glucose levels drop significantly between 2:00 am and 3:00 am, and our bodies respond by releasing hormones that raise blood sugar levels to level them out.

As you can see, our bodies go through a rollercoaster of glucose levels every night! Eating a low-sugar, low GI/GL bedtime snack can prevent our blood sugar levels from dropping too low and lessen the Somogyi effect. This can affect your choices in the morning, because your blood sugar levels won't be as low.

Please know that the point of sharing this information isn't to say that you need a bedtime snack to get through the sugar detox. I acknowledge that there may be a transition time where you might feel that such a snack may help you succeed. If a bedtime snack means that you are less inclined to eat something sugary, then go for it!

Snacks consumed later at night are often eaten in front of the tv or while doing other activities like reading or scrolling through social media. Any time we eat, we need to be mindful of it and pay attention to what we eat and how much. When we are present while we are eating, not only will we make better choices, but we will enjoy our food even more!

Mindful eating is so important that we will take our time to cover the main principles later in this Chapter.

Summary: Healthy bedtime snack is your personal choice. If you feel that a bedtime snack can prevent you from eating something sugary, go for it.

Does the Order in Which I Eat My Food Matter?

No research supports a specific order for each food group to be consumed. However, eating salads at the beginning of the meal may make a difference in how much we eat, likely because we fill our stomachs first with high-fibre, filling food. Our stomachs can only hold so much at once, and starting with a salad is a great way to ensure that we're getting high-fibre, healthy, low GI/GL food into our day. And if we're thinking about our kids, how often do they say that they're too full for vegetables but then often have "room" for dessert? Ensuring that they get their healthy, low GI, high-fibre foods at the beginning of the meal is one way to overcome these excuses!

Summary: There is no scientific proof regarding the order of food that we eat. However, there are obvious advantages to eat the salad first. We ensure that we get high-fibre, healthy, low GI/GL food (especially for kids). And also, salad is a filling food that prevents us from overeating.

MINDFUL AND UNDISTRACTED EATING

When you think of "mindfulness", it may conjure up thoughts of yogis or silent meditation. But you don't need a mountain peak or babbling brook to be mindful - as busy moms, we can be aware of what we're eating without disengaging from what's going on around us. Christopher Willard calls it "informal mindful eating" in his 2019 article "6 Ways to Practice Mindful Eating", Christopher Willard calls it "informal mindful eating". He encourages self-compassion and acknowledgement of distractions that surround us daily; we also need to realize our incredible ability to multitask and be completely capable of being mindful of what we're eating.

Here's a synopsis of Christopher Willard's 2019 guidance in his "6 Ways to Practice Mindful Eating", with my own sugar-focused thoughts interlaced:

1. Eat slowly

If we eat rapidly, we are likely to overeat. We need to slow down and stop eating when our bodies say they're full. Eating slower is one of the best ways to get our mind and body on the same page, communicating what we need as fuel and nutrition. Our bodies send the signal to tell us that we're full (the "satiation signal") about 20 minutes after the brain realizes we're full and tells us to stop eating. This is a major factor behind overeating. However, if you slow your eating down, you allow your body to catch up with your brain, and truly hear the signals about what is enough. A simple way to slow down is to think of what a grandparent may have told you about "proper table manners": sitting down to eat, chewing each bite many times.

2. Learn personal hunger signals

Are you eating because of an emotional want or an actual body need? Our minds and emotions are often the loudest voices when it comes to what we think we need, but being mindful of our situations and emotional state will bring wisdom about what we truly need. The emotional signals will differ for each of us; they could be stress, sadness, frustration, boredom, or even happiness. But instead, let's listen to our bodies; is your energy low, your stomach growling, or are you a bit lightheaded? Instead of eating when our mind tells us to, we need to listen to our bodies. Proper mindful eating is taking the time to listen to our bodies. If you think your body is saying "you need to buy that giant bag of Costco chocolate", you're fooling yourself! So ask yourself what your body's hunger signals are, what your emotional hunger triggers are, and learn how to differentiate between them.

3. Cultivate a mindful kitchen

There is a big difference between eating alone at random times and eating with others at specific times and places. I'm assuming I'm not alone in the fact that my worst food decisions are made at times when I'm alone, it's not mealtime, and/or I'm rushed or responding to some sort of emotional stimulus. One way to eat mindlessly is to wander into and through our kitchens, looking through cabinets, just to see what's there that might fill that empty space or time. Or it might be a random time of day or place, and there's something convenient at the roadside, or we find a chocolate bar in the centre console of our car. We don't need to eat, and we might not even want to eat, but we do... this is the epitome of mindless eating. We need to be proactive about our meals and snacks. Mindless eating is completely unproductive and prevents us from developing healthy environmental cues that tell us what and how much to eat. It also wires our brains and creates new signals (remember how we talked about rewiring the brain in Chapter 1?) for eating that is often far from ideal or healthy. We want to remove (and certainly not create) habits and cues where we think we need sugar whenever we do a certain activity. It's not that we want to eliminate snacking altogether, because as we know from Chapter 1 when we discussed our blood sugar level changes, eating every 3-4 hours is very healthy. But it's best to eat our main meals when we're sitting down at a table at a scheduled time, with others.

Our kitchens should be organized to encourage healthy eating and gathering of healthy food. Think about what you and your family bring into your kitchen and where things are put away. What's more accessible and visible - healthy foods or sugary foods? When food is easy to get, it's easy to eat.

I'm not saying to go overboard and plan out every single bite you put into your mouth. It's important to allow ourselves to enjoy special occasions, and not have anxiety surrounding unplanned moments that should be enjoyed. But we need to be aware that our newly-developed eating habits may change during different times of year or occasions. Being aware is a big part of mindfulness and mindful eating. It's important to know what is happening (eating sugary food on a special occasion) and then let it go and move on and forward to when you can get back to what your habits have become. Being aware of these times when you might be likely to eat something that isn't on the "yes" list will also support you. You will inherently make better choices in those moments, rather than stressing out about them beforehand or during. Those times are for enjoyment, not for over-analyzing each item's GI/GL on the Christmas table. And the longer you live with your low-sugar lifestyle, the easier it will be to recognize what you do and don't want, and more importantly, what you do and don't need.

4. Understand your motivations

This is where we further explore eating food that is emotionally comforting vs. eating nutritionally healthy food. We can find that balance - the balance between nourishing and satisfying and comforting. It might take a bit of rewiring and realizing that we don't need "fake" sugar to be satisfied. When we take the time to enjoy what we're eating based on the taste and what it gives us nutritionally, we are more likely to continue going back to the foods that nourish our bodies. As we move forward with eating healthier, lower-sugar foods, and a greater variety of naturally sweet foods, we will be less likely to binge on processed and added sugars. In turn, we will be more likely to enjoy healthy foods and find them mentally and physically satisfying. And the list of the foods we love and enjoy that check off both of these boxes will grow and grow as we go further and further into our new lifestyle.

5. Connect more deeply with your food

Ok, when I initially read this suggestion, I found it a bit ridiculous. Connect with my food? Should I have a little heart to heart with my apple about how much I appreciate the natural sugars it contains and ask it to provide me with the same satisfaction as the chocolate bar I ignored in the vending machine? Thankfully, this isn't what Willard was talking about. He brought to light the true disconnection we have with our food, unless we're farmers. Most of us don't think twice about where our food comes from, even if we read the packaging and nutritional information (which we've started doing now, right?). It might be hard to connect with a

Hershey's kiss... but an apple... someone planted that seed, tended to that tree, and then after many years an apple grew and was harvested at the perfect time and brought to us to enjoy. It's fascinating when you spend some time thinking about the miracle of a simple piece of fruit and everything that needs to happen perfectly for that fruit to end up in your hand.

Beyond that piece of fruit, we should consider all of the people involved in the meal that ended up on your plate, whether it's the loved ones (or yourself) who took the time to prepare it, or the grocery staff who stocked the produce, and then to those who grow them. Spending time being mindful of the human effort and care involved in what we eat makes it easy to feel grateful and also connected to the food. You can even go so far as to reflect on the cultural traditions that brought you what you're eating and the recipes used to create the delicious dish. This kind of mindfulness supports our success in our lower-sugar lifestyle, because it helps us make better and smarter choices about the processed vs sustainable and natural food we put onto the table for our family and us.

6. Attend to your plate

Again, I read this and had visions of saluting my plate or giving it a bit of extra special polishing. But again, that's not the point. This is key to distracted eating vs. just eating. As we covered already, we don't want to multitask and eat, because this isn't listening to what we need. We'll often end up eating something sugary that only temporarily (or not at all) alleviates what our bodies need. With your next meal, try single-tasking. Try to "just eat". The entire purpose of that space in time is to eat and enjoy what you're eating. What's in front of you on your plate is important not only because it's what's fueling your body. It is important because your family is watching. They learn from you and what you choose to put on your plate (and perhaps their plates), and why it's there. Take the time to talk about the food, where it came from, and why you chose it. Explain the history of the meal, whether it's a "my grandma made something just like this, but I changed it slightly because…" or the cultural story behind the food and where it came from. There is an amazing show for kids on Netflix called "Waffles and Mochi," where 2 characters from a frozen food land come to earth to learn about fresh and delicious food. I recommend it as a way to introduce food to your children. Kids will learn about where food comes from and how it can be made in delicious ways.

Summary: Mindful eating is an essential component in sugar detox preparation. Maybe for us, busy moms, it will be more challenging because we always rush and think more about others than ourselves. Our poor choices for food are made when it is random, unscheduled. So it is worth improving eating because it will help us stop sugar cravings.

You're educated, prepared, and you know what to eat. The Next Step is a Big One. We tackle the actual process of detoxing from sugar. Yes, it's a big step, and I know you can do it. We'll do it together.

4

STEP 4 - DETOX

WHAT IS SUGAR DETOX AND WHAT CAN YOU EXPECT?

There are so many trends that use the term "detox", and they aren't only about health and wellness journeys. We detox from social media, from television and news, from going out too much, or from unhealthy relationships. Have you noticed that when someone says "I'm detoxing from social media", or "I'm detoxing from this unhealthy relationship", those around them are usually very supportive of their decision? It's challenging to overlook the negative effects that these elements have on our lives and mental health.

But you may have noticed that this isn't always the case when we try to "detox" from food. Why is it that when we mention detoxing from a food product like sugar, we are sometimes met with suspicion and a lack of support? It could be two things:

1. A lack of understanding from those who don't understand just how addictive sugar is and how negatively it affects our bodies, or
2. Those who also struggle with their sugar intake don't want to be forced to acknowledge that they can change, perhaps because they're not ready.

This might seem like an obstacle, but it's an incredible launching-off point for you and those in your life. These situations present two opportunities for those of us who are taking this big step to improve ourselves and the lives of others. We can educate those who don't understand, and encourage those who also struggle with their sugar intake. And you are well-equipped to do both now.

Summary: You already learned that processed sugar is unhealthy. Eliminating it from your meals is a huge step forward. Your body and your family with thank you later. No matter what, keep going towards your goals

How is a Sugar Detox Different from a Diet?

As you know, this is not a diet or a plan to focus on "thou shall not". I want you to see all of the amazing things you *can* have and *can* do with my sugar detox 5-step program. This is not a situation where you deny yourself everything you want or reject everything that satisfies you food-wise. This sugar detox plan shows you how to reframe your ideas of sweetness and detox from it. This isn't an instant transformation. It's a life-long commitment.

This book was written by someone like you - a busy mom who wants a clear path to success. This isn't a one-size-fits-all plan or a calculation that doesn't consider you. I am writing this for both of us, because I want you to have what I didn't when I started my wellness journey into being less reliant on sugar.

In this book, we do not put a fixed duration for detox. I will not say that to succeed, you need to stick to a 3-

day, 7-day, or 21-day specific plan; it wouldn't be reasonable for a busy mom whose life changes daily. This is a new approach because none of the books or articles I read when I was looking for answers worked for me. We'll cover the "phases" of detox, where *you* decide what makes the most sense for you and your family. The idea is to set small goals and gradually transition from shorter time periods of removing some sugary food items to longer periods of time. We replace sugary food with other, equally delicious options.

As mentioned, this is a gradual lifestyle change, not a strict diet where on day one you remove every can of soda pop or every single piece of candy or chocolate from your house and burn it by the light of the crescent moon in some sort of cleansing ceremony. While that would be entertaining, it's not reasonable.

This is not a guide on how to become 100% sugar-free all the time; we will continue our lives with holidays, vacations, birthdays, and the sweet food that will come with that. We will, however, have the ability to plan our meals better and make choices that are consistent with our goals and lifestyle. We will also give ourselves grace and understanding when we overindulge. We will get back on track, knowing that we haven't undone all of our good work with one occasion. Our mantra when we realize we're slipping back into old ways or had a bit too many two-bite brownies at the Christmas party is "keep going". And we'll teach our children this mindset too!

Summary: The sugar detox described in this book is a gradual lifestyle change. We still will enjoy occasions and the sweet food that come with them. However, we will learn how to make better choices of food in our daily life.

WHEN TO START THE DETOX

Just as important as the "how" to detox, is the "when". There is not going to be an absolutely perfect time to start the detox, so this isn't a place where I'll offer reasons to put off starting your new lifestyle, because those will always be there!

However, sometimes are not optimal for starting a detox.

When Not to Start

Rather than go through the best times for starting, I'll weed out the less-than-optimal situations for starting a detox:

• **You're stressed more than usual**

If you are trying to manage more stress than usual, this is not the time to start a detox. You need to be in a place of internal peace and have space in your day and mind to take on this challenge.

• **Before a calendar holiday**

Holidays are meant to be enjoyed, and a big part of our holidays (whether we like it or not) is the food. Once you have established your new routine and eating habits, you will be well-equipped to handle the temptations of holidays. But putting yourself in a situation where sweets surround you is just a way to create more struggle than necessary.

• **Before a vacation**

The reason behind this is pretty much the same as for a holiday. It is not the best when you expect to be enjoying yourself, but you would deny yourself the food you truly want. Just like calendar holidays, once you've mastered your reliance on sugar, you will be able to go on vacation like a champ.

• Times of big-life changes for yourself or your family

New jobs, new schools, a new home, a new pet... any of these things take a lot of mental and physical energy, even if you're not the one who is directly going through the change. Wait until things are settled.

See, that's only four points of when not to start! That leaves so many other opportunities to begin your new life.

Summary: It is up to you to decide when to go through a sugar detox. However, it will be easier to go through it when there are no upcoming holidays, vacations, or highly stressful situations.

The Excuse of "I'm Not Ready"

This excuse 100% depends on your mindset, and I can't change your mind. However, we did a lot of work on mindset and getting ourselves ready in Chapter 2, so remember the things that you did and go back and read your goals and remind yourself of your motivational black holes. Know that you have already decided that you are worthy of going through this process.

Also, remember you are what you believe in. If you constantly repeat that you're not going to succeed, you're right. If you constantly repeat that you're "not ready", call yourself out on that nonsense, and ask yourself exactly what "ready" looks like, then. What do you actually need to be "ready"? It's natural to be afraid of failure and not begin something because of this fear. But you are exactly as ready as you'll ever be, right now.

Building on this, let's redefine what failure looks like, and go back to Attitude of Gratitude from Chapter 2, where we talked about having an and being gentle with ourselves. Failure *is not* slipping, or being imperfect, or making mistakes. Failure *is* refusing to continue and staying stuck in those human moments of imperfection. It is not a new concept that being imperfect is inherently human, so you can acknowledge moments that won't be perfect and where you might eat something sugary. But the important thing is to know deep down that this doesn't mean anything beyond that moment. The very next moment is new, and you can get back on track. You're ready.

Summary: You are what you believe in. Simply believe that you are ready, and everything else will follow.

Set Yourself Up for Success

I know we agreed not to go through your entire pantry and throw everything away, and I'm still not asking for that. But to begin detox successfully, you need to remove the immediate and obvious temptations. If you have sugary foods at your desk, in your car, or anywhere else that you typically reach for when you're mindlessly snacking, get rid of them and replace them with other options. Also, as you are preparing your meals, if you come across something in your pantry that is an obvious "high in sugar" item, you can either donate it to a food bank (if it's unopened), or throw it out.

Remember to be mindful while you're eating, and follow the guidelines in Chapter 2. Refer back to that Chapter as much as you need, because the preparation work you did is incredibly important during the detox phase.

Summary: If you need, take a bit more time to work with your mindset. It is the key to success. You CAN do it!

MAKE IT WORK - DETOX

Succeeding in detoxing from sugar will come through tailoring this plan for you, and you've already taken a big step toward that by choosing a plan especially for busy moms.

I highly recommend making/preparing at least 3 days worth of meals and snacks before you start the detox. It will take a time-consuming thing off your plate, and you will not need to think about what you're going to reach for when you want a snack, or what you're going to make for meals. For dinners, you can pre-make slow cooker or pressure cooker "dump meals", where you put all of the ingredients into a large plastic freezer bag, and freeze them. The night before, take the bag(s) out of the freezer and let them thaw in the fridge. In the morning, use a slow cooker or into the pressure cooker when it's time. They're a perfect no-brainer, and you'll be set with your low-sugar meals!

Summary: Preparation is key. It is very simple, but it removes a lot of temptations to eat something sugary.

Create Your Timeline / Phases of Detox

Remember - we're not going cold turkey on all added sugar here, folks. We don't want (or need) to go all crazy-pants on our friends and families because our brains and bodies are completely freaking out, so we're going to create a timeline and phases for a successful, realistic, and manageable detox.

You need to ensure you're realistic about what is achievable. I'm not implying that there is any reason you can't be successful or that you shouldn't push your boundaries and comfort level a bit, but you're a busy mom with a lot on your plate. So, decide right from the start what is reasonable for you, your life, and your family.

I will outline recommendations of the different phases, and you choose what works best for you. If you find that you feel able to move on to the next phase, do so! And if you feel like you need another day or so, take it. Successful completion means moving on to the next phase.

Summary: There will be no strict duration of detox. Only recommendations that you can adapt for yourself. Start with those recommendations and see if it works for you. Next time when you do the detox, increase the duration of each phase and see if it still works. And so on.

Phase 1

This phase is three to five days. You will eliminate the "obvious" added sugar items from your diet. Find out how long you can "survive" without it, and this will be your duration. These are the items where you don't have to read the labels, refer to the GI/GL chart, or think twice about the high-sugar content in these foods. Examples of these are cakes, candies, chocolate, sugary cereals, ice cream, and sugary drinks.

On day one of this phase, if you find this simply too overwhelming and you have one sweet item you rely on the most, eliminate it on day 2 instead. Remember, this is a realistic and long-term lifestyle change. Don't make yourself unnecessarily miserable!

This is the perfect opportunity to start using the Food Swaps chart in Appendix 3. We're starting to train our brains what true and natural sweetness tastes like. You *can* eat sweet things! Remember this. They're just not fake, overly-sweet and processed foods.

Summary: In phase 1, we remove obvious sugar from our diet: cakes, cookies, chocolate, candies, ice cream, sugary cereals and drinks. And you can start using food swaps from Appendix 3 to find out healthy alternatives.

Recommended duration is 3-5 days.

Phase 2

This phase is seven to 21 days. This might seem like a lot of variation, but I can't pretend to know exactly your situation or what's reasonable for you. The final goal is that within that period of time, you will have detoxed from processed sugar!

You've successfully eliminated all of the "obvious" sugary food from your meals and snacks, so now it's time to dive in and use what you've learned so far. In this phase, we will eliminate other sugary food with "hidden" sugars and be very intentional about what we are eating.

This is the time to consider pretty much everything you're eating, and start reading the labels and apply what you learned in Chapter 1. You don't have to do this all at once, though. You can start with one of your regular meals. For example, if you often eat yogurt for breakfast, look at the label and determine how much sugar is in a serving. If you take the time to compare the labels, you will find out many low-sugar yogurt options.

Another example is if you often eat toast or sand-wiches, look at the label to see how much sugar is in a serving. If your current bread is high in sugar, you can decide what other bread you will buy the next time you go to the grocery store, keeping in mind the guidelines in Chapter 3.

Continue doing this evaluation of your food and keeping the amount of sugar under the recommended daily values:

Women: 25 grams = 6 teaspoons
Men: 36 grams = 9 teaspoons
Children (2-18 years old): 24 grams = 6 teaspoons
(American Heart Association Inc, 2019; American Heart Association Inc, n.d.-b)

Once you've done this, you can go further and look into the GI/GL rating of the food for an even better understanding. Being actively involved in the decisions to eat better helps you feel more in control and supports long-term memory of what to look for in the future! Appendix 3 will be a very valuable resource as you swap out your higher sugar food for lower sugar. Also, Appendix 2 has some information you can refer to regarding where food falls on the GI.

We will cover what to do after Phase 2 in the next Chapter, but we'll continue with the actual detox for now.

Summary: In phase 2, we remove "hidden" sugar from our diet.

Start evaluating the food you eat by reading labels. Keep the amount of sugar under recommended:

- for women/kids: 24 g = 6 teaspoons

- for men 36 g = 9 teaspoons

Use Appendix 2 to find out where that food falls in GI/GL. And if the value is high, use Appendix 3 to find out food swaps.

If it is overwhelming, do it gradually and start with a food you eat more often.

Recommended duration is 7-21 days.

MANAGING SUGAR CRAVINGS AND WITHDRAWAL SYMPTOMS DURING DETOX

The biggest challenges that people are facing during sugar detoxification are cravings and withdrawal symptoms. And this is what we will cover now.

Identify Why You Turn to Sugar

Why do we turn to sugar as the thing that solves our problems or rewards us? Whether it's fatigue, stress, or celebration, we need to determine the external triggers that create the response of wanting sugar.

My greatest source of the "external drive" toward sugar started with not eating in a way that properly fueled my body. I didn't eat the slow, natural sugars that would sustain me throughout my day of work, caring for children, cooking, cleaning, and all of the things that come along with being a mom. When I would feel like I was starting to crash, I knew I could get a quick "pick me up" if I ate something sugary. And yes, it worked… for a short time. And then I would crash with fatigue and need more sugar to pick me up again. It was a vicious cycle.

There is no judgement here. We are all doing our best, and you need to give yourself grace and believe that you have been doing the best you can with what you know. But now you've learned something new that will equip you to achieve your life that is free of sugar dependence!

Take some time to think about (and even better if you write it down, because writing things down is key to making them stick in our brains) the last time you really craved sugar. Where were you? Did something happen that affected you emotionally, or did you feel it more like a physical need? Now that we've got the mental and memory juices flowing a bit, try to determine the root cause of why you feel you need processed and refined sugar.

Summary: Take your time to write down:

- When did you eat sugary food last time?

- Why did you eat it?

- Why did you choose it?

- In which situation do you eat it?

We will need those answers later.

Generating the Same Positive Emotional Responses (From Things Other than Sugar)

Food and eating are part of our culture. It's a social thing we do together, and it makes us feel good. Therefore, it's not surprising that so many of us associate food with positive emotions, and that you and I associate sugar with these positive emotions. We already covered how our brains respond to sugar and create a (false) positive feedback loop detrimental to our health. Let's uncover other things that can create the same positive emotional response.

When you think of what is behind the drive to eat sugar, it's about what it does for us emotionally and physically if you take away the taste entirely. We feel energized, focused, more positive, and generally happier. But we don't need sugar for these reactions. It's just a quick fix we've come to associate with sugar.

Summary: Take your answers that you just write down and try to think about what else (not sugar) can generate the same response.

Energy and Focus

Sugar causes that immediate spike that makes us feel like we have more energy, and in essence, we do - but only temporarily. There are better ways to gain energy and to avoid the sugar-related crash. We all know that midday slump. You reach for something quick and easy to get that boost, but try these things proposed by Fisher in the 2020 article "5 Ways to Beat the Midday Slump Without Sugar (or Coffee)" instead:

1. Move your body

"Small doses of physical activity have actually been shown to be more effective in boosting energy than caffeine in sleep-deprived women. So when you hit a wall, spend 10 minutes walking around the block or up and down the stairwell, or even finding a corner to do jumping jacks and pushups."

2. Refresh-mint

"Studies have shown that the smell of peppermint can lessen fatigue and increase mental alertness. Have a cup of peppermint tea, pop a piece of strong gum or mint..."

3. Fuel properly with good fats

"Fat also happens to be the most energy-efficient fuel source for the body, and provides a sustained boost that won't leave you crashing. Good fat sources to consume mid-afternoon include avocado, macadamia nuts, or any type of nut butter paired with fruit."

4. Get your protein in

"A snack rich in protein will help fuel you through the afternoon and provide stable energy..."

Summary: Above are just a few examples of what can give you the same response as sugar.

Positivity and Happiness

You might have moments where you think you're missing out by not eating sugar, and this might make you feel a bit down. Yes, sugar may have even felt like a trusted friend you knew you could count on to make you feel better about yourself. But of course, we already know that sugar is a fickle friend and is not a reliable source of comfort or happiness, and we are looking for true joy that comes from within and not from what we eat. Here are some better ways to improve your mood:

1. Get outside

Breathing in some fresh air, listening to water cascading over rocks, watching leaves dance, and gardening are proven ways to improve mood. Many of us are missing connection to the earth, and even short periods of time in nature are incredible mood boosters.

2. Call a friend

True connection with someone we know who cares for us produces those warm, happy, fuzzy feelings that just aren't sustainable with sugar.

3. Let's get physical

Yes, exercise improves mood, but I'm referring to touch in this case, like petting an animal or hugging someone you love. The beneficial emotional flood that results from the sensation of touch is scientifically proven and is better than a chocolate bar any day.

4. Meditate

Focusing and quieting your mind in moments of over-whelm and stress can break your reliance on consuming sugar and other external sources of positivity. Taking the time to be mindful of what you are grateful for and appreciating what you have can bring immense and undeniable happiness that cannot be taken away.

Summary: Above are some more examples of what can give you the same response as sugar.

Response to Low-Sugar Lifestyle

I know we already discussed how sugar affects your body and brain in Chapter 1. Here we will dive into what happens when we teach our bodies something new and different from what it's used to.

Our bodies are creatures of habit, and they like it when things are the same, and things don't happen suddenly. This is one of the big reasons why my sugar detox process is gradual - we don't want to freak our bodies out! However, our bodies are stubborn, even if something is bad for us. Our bodies like consistency.

As our bodies adapt to a lower-added-sugar diet and we eat sugar less frequently, the symptoms of detox and our cravings will be less intense and less persistent. Some symptoms might be worse at certain times of day, like between meals or at night before bed (Santos-Longhurst, 2020). Also, if we have built up habits of eating our sugary food, like the mid-afternoon slump at work, while we're waiting for our kids to do activities or driving, those might bring on symptoms and cravings.

Summary: Every person has habits, including bad ones, and does not like sudden changes. That is why the current sugar detox program is a gradual process. Our body and brain will adapt slowly to our new low-sugar lifestyle, and detox symptoms and cravings will occur less and less.

How Our Body Will Respond

You may have considered or even tried a strict detox where you cut sugar (or something else) out of what you eat immediately and completely. You likely found that this kind of immediate removal (especially something we're addicted to, like sugar) can cause physical issues.

How our bodies will react will be different for everyone - it will depend on factors like current stress levels, how well-rested we are, and how much sugar we ate before the detox. According to Juliana Roman's 2018 article titled "Seven stages of sugar withdrawal (And why it's all worth it!)", you can expect the following stages, which I've adapted slightly:

1. Well, this seems pretty easy

When you first start detoxing from sugar, your body hasn't figured out that this is what you're doing. It hasn't yet registered that you're not pumping a bunch of added sugar into the brain. However, you'll think this is a walk in the park with your food swaps and prepared meals and snacks!

2. Here come the cravings

As we know, sugar addiction is serious and not one to be taken lightly, and your brain and body aren't going to let it go without a fight. You may even have dreams about giving into cravings and eating all the sweets you want. But stay the course, you can do it! Eat your pre-chosen snacks, and fill your plate with protein and high-fibre foods. You've got this, keep your eye on the prize!

3. Getting ahead of yourself

The prize will come, and you can overcome obstacles. Similar to when people stop drinking coffee and have headaches, sugar withdrawal commonly causes headaches too. You might feel dizzy and have a hard time focusing, or feel generally unwell. Drink lots of water, get some fresh air, and consider aromatherapy oils that help with headaches like peppermint, rosemary, lavender, eucalyptus, or a blend. You can do it, and everything worth achieving comes with effort.

4. Aches and pains

Your body may feel achy and sore, perhaps even like you've got the flu. In this case, take some time to pamper yourself, and try having a warm bath with Epsom salts (studies suggest this may help flush out toxins). But I'm not a doctor - if you feel unwell or out of sorts, get checked out by your physician.

5. The swinging moods

Your brain has figured out that you're denying it the sugar that it's used to, and it is screaming for it. It's normal to expect that if you're not feeling great, you're going to have some mood swings, and we already know the effect that all of our added sugar has on our "reward system" in the brain. We'll help you get through this in our Facebook group. Link to it you can find at the end of this book.

6. Feeling shaky

Some people get "the shakes". These mild tremors can be linked to stress and lower blood sugar, so if you feel shaky, try having a snack or even some herbal tea. If you're worried about the shaking, see your doctor.

7. Coming out the other side

Suddenly, you'll realize that you feel pretty good. In fact, you feel better than ever, and you aren't craving sugar. It could take a few days or a few weeks, but you'll understand why you started this process. You'll feel more clear-headed, brighter, and happier, and each day will get easier and easier. You no longer have the over-whelming cravings that drove you to eat sugar before. You've improved your health both short and long term, and don't have the slumps throughout the day due to the blood sugar roller coaster you were on before.

Summary: During sugar detox, your body will go through 7 stages that we mentioned above. Some stages are challenging.

Join our Facebook group and find support from people who are doing the same thing. The link to the group can be found at the end of the book.

How Our Brain Will Respond

Beyond physical symptoms of eating less sugar, we can also expect our minds to have an opinion about taking away something that's changing the way the brain works.

To refresh your memory from Chapter 1, sugar acts on the part of our brain that makes us feel good, and causes a release of dopamine, the hormone that is linked to our "reward system". Our reliance on sugar means that we need to rewire our brains to accept rewards from elsewhere, and for a little while, our brains will revolt at not getting what they want.

Once we've removed our reliance on sugar and go through the steps in this book, we can expect to have more consistent energy levels, more stable moods, a better appreciation of our food, and a better relationship with what we're eating.

However, to get to that point, we will likely need to go through a few less comfortable things. I've adapted and added to some of the symptoms outlined in the 2020 article "What Is a Sugar Detox? Effects and How to Avoid Sugar" by Santos-Longhurst:

- **Anxiety**

You may feel anxious, nervous, restless, or irritable, or as though you are less patient or "on the edge". You are irritated with your new routine, you might think: "Sugar detox is not easy", "I cannot do that". Or you can start worrying more about tomorrow: "How will I do that tomorrow?"

• Changes in sleep patterns

Occasionally, those who detox from sugar report problems with sleep. This could be due to not having that "sugar crash" that essentially forces you to sleep.

• Cognitive issues

It may feel like you're having difficulty concentrating, or you keep forgetting things. It might feel like you're struggling with staying on task in places like work or school.

• Cravings

We've already touched on craving sugar, but you may find that you're starting to crave other foods, especially simple and processed carbohydrates like white bread, white pasta, and potato chips. This is because your body is smart... it knows that there can be a high amount of sugars in these foods - just check out the GI/GL rating of the foods you're craving to get some insight! Craving another food is a good sign because you are re-training your brain. Just make sure that this replacement is healthier.

- **Depressed mood**

Some people report feeling "down", which can be due to the decreased instant dopamine release from eating added sugar. You feel sad every time you "slip", you are losing interest to a lower-sugar lifestyle.

There are some challenges on your sugar detox journey. How to cope with them we will discuss right away.

Summary: Not only your body but also your brain will revolt sugar detox. But you will overcome that and adapt to a new reality with time.

How to Cope With the Side Effects

Don't let these temporary and inconvenient symptoms derail you. You're perfectly equipped for success, and your commitment to the end goal will propel you.

Your "Why"

Identify your "why" if you haven't already done this. It can be one thing, it can be three things, but not more than three, because beyond 3 things, our brains have a harder time remembering them, and it also dissolves their level of importance in our memory. If it helps you, write them down on sticky notes and put them throughout your house.

Mantra

If it helps, your mantra for when you're struggling with side effects could be "This too shall pass". Often a mantra can be helpful when we are struggling mentally with uncomfortable situations. Here are some other options of things you can say to yourself when you're struggling:

- "I am strong. I am capable. I am worthy of a healthier life."
- "I have everything I need to get through this."
- "I deserve to be better. I can be better."
- "My goal is within reach. This feeling won't stop me."

Visualization

Visualization can help, too. If you feel the cravings too much, the side effects intolerable, or where you're feeling especially tempted to eat something sugary, do this:

1. Go somewhere quiet, or put on headphones to block out any background noise.

2. **Breathe.** Pay attention to your breath. Hold a deep breath for 3 seconds. Exhale completely through your mouth, making an "ahhhh" sound as you exhale. Focus on your breathing. Do this 10 times.

3. **Picture yourself putting away the moment you're struggling with.** If it's a situation, picture the scene. If it's a specific food, picture it. Putting these away could look a number of ways:

- Writing or drawing your tough spot on a blackboard, and erasing it.
- The picture of your tough spot is 3D in paper form in front of you, and the size of it corresponds to how greatly it is affecting you. Visualize yourself crumpling or folding up this paper, and putting it into a wooden box. Put a large lock on the box. If this issue is one that you need to deal with later, put the box aside, or entrust it to someone else - be it a friend, family member, or God (or the higher power that speaks to you). If you don't need to deal with the situation later, throw the entire box into a large fire.
- Visualize your tough spot as a balloon, and either pop the balloon or let it go and watch it disappear into the sky.

Do Something Else

Doing something else is an excellent method for getting through side effects and cravings. If you're sitting on the couch watching tv and are experiencing withdrawal symptoms, get up and do something else. Physically moving yourself from a space in which you are feeling discomfort can trick your mind into leaving the discomfort in that space. Play a card game, organize your books or collections, look through pictures of your family, go for a walk... do something different and distract your brain.

Food Can Help with Side Effects and Cravings

Yes, there is food that can help you through the detox phases! We have already covered the best food to eat in our lower-sugar lifestyle. Here is a summary of the main points.

1. Avoid added sugar

We emphasize one more time that we want to reduce added or refined sugar that you can find in processed food and desserts. Natural sugar refers to fruits (or vegetables) in their natural state, as they are in the field or garden.

2. High-fibre foods

Fibre promotes feelings of being full and prevents overeating, helps stabilize sugar levels.

3. Lots of water

Start replacing soft drinks and other sugary drinks with water. Just this step alone is a huge improvement in your routine. When you feel hunger drink water first. You might notice that sometimes you are confused between thirst and hunger.

4. Protein-rich food

Protein reduces appetite. It takes longer to digest protein food. That is why you will feel full for a longer time. There are 2 main types of protein: animal and plant-based, so it will fit your current diet if you are vegetarian.

According to the 2018 article "Does your Gut Help Control Food Cravings?" by Donna Schwenk, the microbes in our stomach could be a great contributor to our cravings for sugar. And one of the fastest ways to help this is to give your body extra minerals and cultured foods. And to avoid what happens when we eat sugar - our body and brain screaming "more!", we can add the following to our meals and snacks:

5. Cultured / Fermented vegetables

Either store-bought or homemade, fermented vegeta bles are powerful ways to help your stomach microbes. They also support your immune system with their high levels of B and C vitamins.

6. Kefir

This fermented milk or non-dairy drink is much stronger than yogurt with cultured probiotics with over 50 strains of beneficial microbes. It also has a lot of B and C vitamins, and helps absorb nutrients from the other food we eat. You can add kefir to a smoothie as a great way to integrate it into your day.

7. Prebiotics

These specialized plant fibres are what feed the benefi- cial stomach microbes. If you are craving juice, why not juice some low GI/GL food and give your stomach that soluble fibre to help control your cravings? Some of the best sources of prebiotics are low GI berries, broccoli, leeks, kale, bananas, nuts, and seeds.

Here's a list of some other food/ingredients to consider that might help with your sugar cravings:

8. Caraway seeds

Research suggests adding caraway seed to your diet can help regulate blood sugar levels. Also, caraway seeds are a great source of fibre, which we already know has a beneficial effect on blood sugar and feelings of fullness (Link, 2019).

9. Frozen grapes

A great substitute for when you're craving ice cream, frozen grapes give natural sweetness with the consistency of tiny mouthfuls of frozen sorbet. Taking time to eat them very slowly and enjoy the sweetness of each one is especially helpful (Brown West-Rosenthal, 2017).

10. Plant-based fats

Avocado is an excellent way to add a creamy texture to our food while increasing the nutrients and healthy fats. Also, coconut oil (paired with a dash of cinnamon) can provide the sense of eating sugars from the natural sweetness (Brown West-Rosenthal, 2017).

Summary: Here are some ways to cope with the side effects of sugar detox:

- Remember your "WHY" and keep going.
- Encourage yourself by repeating your "MANTRA".
- Visualize how you cope with your problem.
- Do something else.
- Pick a food you like from the list above and include it in your menu.

You're not an island, alone in this journey and only taking yourself into consideration. You're also not alone *on* an island (although don't we sometimes wish we were?), so we're going to bring our family along with us on our journey.

I'm not implying that your children need to go through the sugar detox phases - the one thing you certainly don't need while you're navigating the withdrawal symptoms is managing a tiny army of humans who are going through the same thing! However, you'll be setting the example and also slowly eliminating the added sugar products from your children's lives too. Having your entire family move toward this healthier lifestyle together means you will have less temptations in your home, and you're getting healthier together!

Before you start the detox, I recommend talking to your family about your decision so they're not surprised and understand what you're doing and why you're doing it. Take the time to educate them (at a level they can understand) about what sugar is and what it can do to their bodies, and how there are better options. Ensure that they are as prepared as you are for this big change, and get them excited for the journey!

Summary: While you will go through a sugar detox, your family will see changes in the grocery you buy and the meals you cook. Talk to them on the level they understand and explain what you will do before you start actual detox.

Advertising Doesn't Help

We briefly covered the advertising of sugary products in Chapter 1, and the ridiculous amount of time and money that food producers spend on making sugar appealing. If the companies that make the food can cause a sugar addiction in children, they've got customers for life.

The food and beverage industry sees our children as a major market force - that is, they actually make decisions on and have influence over what is purchased. Because of this, they are targeted aggressively with an enormous amount of advertising in every area of their lives. There is evidence of product placement and sales tactics on television, in-school marketing, kids clubs, the internet, and even toys and products. There is an unsettling similarity between this advertising toward children and those used by the tobacco industry (Story & French, 2004).

It is proven that children request food items when exposed to them through television and whether they're available in the home (Story & French, 2004). Gradually replacing added sugar food with healthier alternatives and having age-appropriate conversations with our children is an excellent way to get them on board with our new lifestyle. We can't protect them from all advertising sources, but we can educate them and help them think about what they're eating and drinking, and whether it provides what their bodies need.

Summary: Educate your kids about sugar as early as you can. You can not protect them from advertisements. But you can be an excellent example to follow. If your kids still do not talk, they still watch you and remember what mom is eating.

Provide Options at Every Meal

We're committed to bringing our families along on our journey of being healthier, and we believe that this is the best thing for them and us. However, our children might not be quite so quick to jump onto this bandwagon, even if you've spent the time explaining things to them.

A great way to make the transition easier is to make sure that there is one thing on their plate that they will like at every meal. I'm not saying to put candy or sugar-added food on their plate, but if you know that they will always eat something like buttered toast, provide that, and let them have more if they want to. Often children, especially young children, need to be exposed to new foods, flavours, and textures a few times before they're willing to try them. Explain what the food does for them in terms they can understand. For example, you could say that meat has protein that helps them build strong muscles, or vegetables have vitamins that help their brains work better.

Providing options at every meal when serving something new shows your children that you're still considering them, and not forcing them only to eat things they don't like (or don't know that they like!).

Instead of forcing your children to eat something, you could say that you want them to taste it, even just sticking out their tongue to get the flavour. But if you want them to buy into this process and not resent it (or you), don't force them to eat the new food. Don't give in and allow them to eat whatever they want. It's not terrible for them to be a bit hungry, and they know they will eat again soon. It's a fine balance and a bit of a dance to encourage them toward a healthier lifestyle, and some children will be excited about the challenge, and others will be more hesitant. Be patient with them, and keep talking about all of the positive things that will come out of it. You can even make them a part of the times you reward yourself, saying that you'll do something special together as a reward for your new healthier lifestyle!

Summary: Do not force your kids to eat specific food. To make the transition to healthier options, always provide choice. And continue to educate them and be a great example.

Do not Call Sugar "Bad"

Do you remember the food you weren't allowed to eat as a child? I have a feeling that you were likely told that sugary foods were "bad" or something that you were forced to limit, and perhaps you weren't even allowed to try them.

The thing about calling something "bad" to a child is that they will inherently do 2 things with this "bad" thing:

1. They think that it's "bad" and **want it even more**.
2. They believe that there is some shame surrounding that thing called "bad", and then they **start to do it in secret**.

Be careful with children and not teach them that any food is bad. Instead, explain why some choices are better. We need to stop associating certain food with certain body types, as well, because there are many conditions beyond food intake that affect how bodies look.

Summary: We can help prevent our children from becoming addicted to sugar. However, it is better not to teach kids that some food is "bad". Instead, we can explain to them that some choices are better than others.

By now, you have learned about sugar detox stages and what to expect during this journey. You might ask what to do after detox is done? And we will cover an answer to this question in the next Chapter.

5

STEP 5 - NOW WHAT? HOW DO I MAKE IT STICK?

You're prepared. You're pumped. And you're feeling positive about the fantastic life changes you're going to make. You're going to reduce the amount of sugar you eat and remove your reliance on it to get you through the day. You've got a list of delicious food swaps you can refer to whenever you're having a craving or are looking for how to make your sugar intake lower. You even know how to do the detox and have some excellent resources to get through it and succeed.

I'm going to be honest with you - this might not be the only time you go through the detox process. If it is, fantastic! If it's not, it's completely acceptable. The first detox is always the hardest, and even if you were able to reduce how much sugar you eat a little bit, be gratefull Buy yourself flowers and be proud of your progress. No matter how small the steps, moving forward is still moving toward a goal and worth being proud of. Use your experience to figure out what worked best and what can work better for you and your family. Do not give up, and see every successful step as a complete success. Pay attention to how your body feels after even small changes and spend time being grateful for your commitment and those positive effects.

Summary: Be proud of every single step you did toward sugar detox. It does not matter how big or small it is.

So...

WHAT DO YOU DO AFTER DETOX?

At the beginning of the book, we mentioned that diets might have good results while you're actively dieting and following the regimented process. Still, often we're left without a follow-up as they don't explain or outline what to do after. And most often, if/when we stop following the exact steps outlined and try to figure out how to implement what we learned into our "normal" lives, we gradually end up back where we started.

But this book is different. I have a completely different approach to sugar detox because, as you've read over and over, this is a lifestyle, not a diet. This sugar detox does not have a fixed duration. And the "secret" is that **if you want to maintain your results, low-sugar meals should be part of your lifestyle**. And if you are reading this and thinking that maintaining this kind of eating for the rest of your life isn't something you can do, keep reading.

I'm not saying you should stay away from sugar for the rest of your life. I am encouraging you to look into your current eating habits and improve them so that YOU can maintain them.

So here is your after-detox plan:

1. What did you feel after phases 1 & 2?

Write down what you felt after phases 1 & 2. What did you think was easily incorporated into your life and something you can continue doing without effort? What was challenging? The stuff that was simple to do will be incorporated into your daily life. With more complicated items, you will continue working on step 3.

Also, it is crucial to listen to your body. Try to feel the difference in your body after you are eating healthy vs unhealthy. For example, when you eat a cookie and when you eat an apple, your body will thank you for the apple. While the cookie might provide instant gratification, you'll eventually have a sugar crash. At one point, you will start to see the difference. And you will see that your body is thankful for the good stuff.

Here are some notes from my experience:

In phase 1, it was effortless for me to give up soda, sugary drinks, and juices. I was able to replace that with water, water with lemon, tea with mint (without sugar), and compote from frozen fruits (without sugar). I found it more challenging to swap other "obvious" sugar. But because it was just for 3 days, I did it.

In phase 2, it was effortless for me to swap bread for pita, fruit yogurt for plain yogurt with fresh or frozen fruits, cereals for plain oats, and salad dressing and ketchup for homemade alternatives.

But I had difficulties maintaining the results I achieved in phase 1, especially with chocolate. I was able to "survive" without it for 5 days, and did not consider this a failure. In fact, I had improved 5-fold! Before I started the detox, I ate chocolate every day, but now it was every 5th day. I thought that was pretty fantastic! But I put chocolate into my list of things to improve.

2. Design a lifestyle YOU can maintain

By lifestyle, I mean something that you can do daily, plus a few occasions when you can have some exceptions.

I will continue with my example: I have 2 small kids, and I don't want to keep them away from sweets for holidays and birthdays. I still want to enjoy deserts occasionally and especially during vacation. My entire family enjoys eating fresh fruits so much that it is an everyday essential for us. As you can see, sugar is still allowed in my family, and we are not aiming to be completely sugar-free. So, this is our lifestyle. This is what we can stick to.

Think about the lifestyle that YOU can maintain.

3. Pick one thing and improve it

Have a look at the list of challenges you wrote after phases 1 & 2. Analyze the current situation and think about how you can make it better. Set your goal to improve one thing every day. And if something requires more days, then work on it as needed.

It was evident for me to work on my chocolate consumption. However, I was not ready to swap chocolate with fruits. Instead, I changed milk chocolate with dark (75% cocoa) chocolate with less sugar.

4. Add something new to your menu/lifestyle

Of course, to have results, you need gradual changes. Use strategies that we covered in the book:

• Plate template. Make sure you are adjusting your current plate.
• Food lists. Include more or introduce something new from one of the following lists:

  • Filling food
  • Food scientifically proven to burn fat
  • Food that can help with the side effect of detox and cravings

• Drink more water.
• Continue to work with your mindset.
• Improve your discipline. Always prepare food and snacks ahead of time.
• Practice mindful eating.

In my case, I started to eat more filling food: oats, Greek yogurt, and beans. Also, I increased the amount of protein (chicken and cottage cheese) and water. Once I incorporated these swaps and increased my protein, I felt it was easier to replace milk chocolate with dark chocolate, and a homemade "ice cream" made with a frozen banana and cocoa powder. I still eat dark chocolate once a month, but this is already closer to my goal to leave it just for occasions.

5. Review and repeat

In step 3, we picked just one thing to work with. And in step 4, we did not change everything at once. However, our "to do" list is big, so we will move to the next item and repeat steps 3 & 4. At one point, you might go back to step 2 and make changes to your lifestyle as well.

When you feel that you can repeat the detox itself, do it. You can even challenge yourself a little bit more. Next time you do the detox, increase the duration of phases by one day.

The biggest challenge I am working on is replacing processed sugar with natural sugar. Chocolate was not the only item I needed to work with. So, I will keep going. When I finish that, I will work on eliminating any sugar gradually. But I am not aiming for zero sugar in my life, because I believe the body still needs some natural sugar for essential processes.

Summary: Even after detox, we continue to work on improvements to our lifestyle. Seeing your detox from sugar as a lifestyle is a key to maintaining results. Only YOU can decide how your lifestyle will look like. You can reevaluate where you're at and how things are working for you, make adjustments and make it fit your life better.

HOW TO GET BACK ON TRACK AFTER OCCASIONS?

If holidays or vacations are long (at least one week), I suggest going through sugar detox again afterward and repeating phases 1 & 2. If possible, during your "occasion," add a little bit more physical activity. I am not necessarily talking about going to the gym (but you can if that's your thing); I'm just referring to moving your body more in any way you enjoy. For example, every morning, if you are on vacation, take an extra walk along the beach, or participate in beach Zumba or volleyball. In wintertime, go outside and play with your kids. I am sure they will keep you busy for a while. If it is too cold, have a dancing party inside.

And I believe that after completing detox and "after-detox", the next "occasion" you will more easily manage your desire to eat sweets. And probably you will be able to say "no" to some of them. Just look at this like at your chance to eat more tropical fruits or other fruits that you cannot often buy on your regular days.

If it is just a one-day birthday party, only buy the sweet food that you need for that day. It is safer to run out of sweets at the party than to have a bunch of leftovers that will tempt you. One day is one day, and you will be sure that there is nothing in your house to tease you the next day. Better to buy a bit more fruits and rely on them. Do not forget to pre-purchase healthy food from the list of food that will help you manage cravings.

And as always, keep in mind your "WHY". It will help you to stay on track.

Summary: It is human nature to want something that is forbidden. So, allow yourself "occasional" sweet treats according to your lifestyle. After a long vacation, repeat detox. After a one-day event, ensure that nothing is teasing you the next day and have healthy alternatives instead.

REWARD YOURSELF

What is something that you would love and that would feel like a real "treat". No, not sugar, something else! Perhaps you'd love a manicure, or a night away, to take a yoga class, or there's a piece of art you've wanted for a long time. It could be anything, and the rewards will be personal and varied, so take some time to think about what would help motivate you through the detox process.

Remember that "reward centre" in the brain that we're retraining to respond to things other than sugar? This is one way we're going to activate it and get the neurons firing for something other than sugar. When we focus on a reward for effort, it creates new synapses - the "small pocket of space between two cells where they can pass messages to communicate" (Sukel, 2019) - in our brains that relate positive outcomes to something other than sugar. Isn't it amazing how we can essentially rewire our brains to support our healthier lifestyle? And as you might remember, this information is stored for the future, so our brains will continue to associate eating less sugar with positive outcomes.

Summary: We will continue to train our brains to associate eating less sugar with positive outcomes.

The "Strategy of Treats"

While those who love sugar automatically associate the word "treat" with "sweet", this concept doesn't mean that at all. Many strategies can work well to help support changing habits or what we eat, but creating a "treat" for a reward at the end can be really fun.

As busy moms who admittedly rely on sugar more than we'd like to, let's completely reframe and redefine what the word treat means to us. I'm willing to bet that most think of the word treat and consider it unhealthy or almost shameful. Why can't we "treat ourselves" and be proud of both the accomplishment and the reward?

Please think of how positively this could impact our children! Let's reframe the concept of treats and make them not about sugar or food at all. This is taking a huge step toward promoting healthy eating and competent eating, especially for our children.

A treat is something that we are grateful for, that brings joy and pleasure into our lives, and that we don't feel guilty about. Treat is a great way to overcome depression and add some "surprises" to a daily routine. Everyone can have different treats, but this is normal. Here is my own list:

- Taking a hot bath
- Swimming
- Spend some time in the spa
- Using scented candles
- Smelling flowers
- Visiting gardening center
- Going to a botanical garden
- Picnic with family
- Walking in the forest
- Skating
- Taking a nap
- Dancing with my daughter
- Listening to birds in the morning
- Walking bare feet on the grass
- Taking a sunbath
- Buying crystals
- Decorating house
- Watching comedy
- Looking photo albums
- Take a massage
- Reading a paper book

Take the time to write down what you consider a treat for yourself and your family. If you need a little extra motivation, you can look at this list and add it. And because nothing on this list will take us off track, feel free to use as many as you need!

Summary: Redefine your definition of treats. Exclude sugar as a treat. And think about what else can give you pleasure and joy.

MAKE THE TIME - BUSY MOMS HAVE BUSY LIVES

We're all busy, and the word "busy" is a response and excuse and way of living. I am not discounting that we are busy moms (check out the title of this, after all!), but I believe we will make time for it if something is important.

Succeeding needs to be a priority to you. You need to believe that:

- You need to make changes and need to address the amount of sugar you eat,
- You want a better life for yourself and your family,

• You are worth it

When someone says that they're "too busy" for something, it just means that it doesn't rank high enough on their priority list to attend to it.

Summary: Always remember that if something is important for you, you will find a time to do it.

SUCCESS IS A FAMILY THING

As mentioned before, I recognize that we don't live in a bubble or on an island as busy moms. To succeed, it's important to follow the steps in the previous Chapter where we talk about how to incorporate your family into this process of healthier living.

You will be setting an incredibly positive outlook on eating and sugar specifically. As you go through this process together as a family, you'll hold each other up and encourage each other.

If they haven't already, your children will start to ask questions about why things are eaten, what's on their plate, and what they see other families eating. A great way to address this is to use the phrase "in our family…". It's a positive and non-judgmental way for your children to stay competent eaters and realize that every family is different, and that's ok. For example, your child might come home from school and say, "My friend always gets a donut in their lunch. I like donuts too. It's not fair that I always have an apple". Your response could be, "In our family, we believe that nature provides us with the best choices, and we value natural sweetness over sugary sweetness. How about we have a donut this weekend?". This way, you're not saying that donuts are bad, but you're reinforcing the education surrounding healthy eating. Also, by offering a donut later, you show that they can be eaten in moderation. This helps kids become competent eaters and not feel like any food is a shameful thing.

Our children are watching us, even when we don't think they are. They are absorbing more than we'll ever realize. And this doesn't change when it comes to our relationship with food. I didn't realize what my children saw until they could talk, and what they said about my eating habits was a bit upsetting. Their comments about what I ate (a lot of sugary foods) and how they wanted it too were a catalyst to figuring out how to change and then writing this book.

Summary: When you start practicing a low-sugar lifestyle for the entire family, your kids will ask you questions about food. Remember not to say that some food is "bad". Instead, use "in our family," we believe that nature gives us the best choices. And all families are different, and it is ok.

FINAL NOTES ON SUCCESS AND SUSTAINABILITY IN THIS PLAN

Thank you for making it so far, and thank you for investing in yourself and your family! Beyond all of the information in this book, I need to summarize some very key points.

- Guarantee of your success is not just one specific thing; it is a combination of what you have already learned, planned, and will achieve through this book.
- "Sugar Detox for Busy Moms" is not a quick fix. This is a lifestyle.
- Faltering isn't failure - you only fail when you give up.

- When you falter, go back to the start, and go back to your plan. Your success lies in your ability to make this plan work for you over and over again.
- Believing in yourself will skyrocket your chances for success.

Summary: I believe in you! YOU and your family can detox from sugar!

Leave a Review!

I would be incredibly thankful if you could take 60 seconds to write a brief review of this book on Amazon, even if it is just a few sentences! Every review counts!

Today you will give back to me, but tomorrow somebody else will give back to you. This is one of the laws of the Universe: the more you give, the more you receive. Let's help each other!

To leave the review scan the QR code below:

Or visit this link:
www.olenasieger.com/sugar-detox-for-busy-moms-reviews

Thank you!

CONCLUSION

I cannot believe our journey is coming to an end! But for YOU, it is just the beginning. And here is your final summary of the action plan.

1. Educate yourself

You finished this step and are ready to use the principles and strategies to achieve sugar detox.

2. Mindset and motivation

It is the most crucial step. You should be 100% sure of your success and have strong motivation and realistic goals. Motivation will keep you on track for the entire journey. The easiest way to start working on that is to practice the morning routine (free download is available on the "Thank you" page) and evening rituals (covered in Chapter 2).

3. Plan meals ahead and enjoy them

Preparation is the key. You should know what you will be eating for several days. Plan before you go to do the grocery.

4. Detox

Use strategies that we covered in different chapters:

- Know your approximate daily sugar intake and keep it under the recommended value (for women/kids: 24 g = 6 teaspoons, for men 36 g = 9 teaspoons),
- Work on most sugary items from your grocery list: swap them for food with lower GI/GL or exclude them when you are ready,
- Use a plate template for every meal,
- Prepare your meals and snacks ahead,
- Use food lists from the book (filling food, low-sugar food, food scientifically proven to burn fat, food that can help with the side effect of detox and cravings),

- Drink more water,
- Find out what generates the same emotions as sugar and use it the next time you have a craving.

5. Maintain results

Design a lifestyle that you can stick to. Gradually improve it as you go. Celebrate your wins. As a treat, use something else, not sugar.

And you are done! As a pleasant "side effect" of sugar detox, you will have weight loss and a healthier lifestyle.

YOU CAN DO IT!

DO NOT FORGET ABOUT FREE GIFT!
JUST FOR YOU!

5 Weird Morning Rituals
That Will Help You to Lose Weight.

Discover "Missing Ingredient"
in Weight Loss Programs.

Scan the QR code below:

Or visit this link:
www.olenasieger.com/5-weird-morning-rituals-to-
lose-weight

JOIN OUR FACEBOOK GROUP!

It is essential to know that you are not alone in your journey. Many moms are going through the same and have the same challenges. Let's support each other by sharing experiences, success stories, simple recipes, positive vibes. Get your questions answered, find friends and have fun.

**Here is our Facebook community.
Scan the QR code below:**

Or visit this link:
https://www.facebook.com/groups/weight.loss.for.
busy.mom

APPENDIX 1

Different names of sugar
(Gameau, 2015)

Agave Nectar	Barbados Sugar	Barley Malt
Beet Sugar	Blackstrap Molasses	Brown Rice Syrup
Brown Sugar	Buttered Sugar	Buttered Syrup
Cane Juice Crystals	Cane Juice	Cane Sugar
Caramel	Carob Syrup	Caster Sugar
Coconut Sugar	Corn Sweetener	Corn Syrup
Corn Syrup Solids	Confectioner's Sugar	Crystal Line Fructose
Date Sugar	Derma Sugar	Dextran
Diastatic Malt	Diastase	Ethyl Maltol
Evaporated Cane Juice	Fructose	Fruit Juice Concentrate
Galactose	Golden Sugar	Golden Syrup
Grape Sugar	High Fructose Corn Syrup	Honey
Invert Sugar	Icing Sugar	Lactose

Malt Syrup	Maltodextrin	Maltose
Maple Syrup	Molasses Syrup	Muscovado Sugar
Organic Raw Sugar	Oat Syrup	Panela
Panocha	Rice Bran Syrup	Rice Syrup
Sorghum	Sorghum Syrup	Sucrose
Sugar	Syrup	Treacle
Tapioca Syrup	Turbinado Sugar	Yellow Sugar

APPENDIX 2

Glycemic Index (GI), Glycemic Load (GL) of some food

Foster-Powell, K., Holt, S. H., & Brand-Miller, J. C. (2002). International table of glycemic index and glycemic load values: 2002. The American Journal of Clinical Nutrition, 76(1), 5–56. https://doi.org/10.1093/ajcn/76.1.5

Adapted and reproduced by permission of Oxford University Press on behalf of the American Society for Nutrition.

Food	Glycemic index (glucose = 100)	Serving size, g	Glycemic load per serving
BAKERY PRODUCTS			
Banana cake, made without sugar	55 ± 10	60	16
Croissant (Food City, Toronto, Canada)	67	57	17
Waffles, Aunt Jemima (Quaker Oats)	76	35	10
BREADS			
100% barley flour bread (Canada)	67	30	9
Bagel, white, frozen (Lender's Bakery, Montreal, Canada)	72	70	25
Baguette, white, plain (France)	95 ± 15	30	15
Corn tortilla (Mexican)	74 ± 7	50	12
Hamburger bun (Loblaw's, Canada)	61	30	9
Pita bread, white (Canada)	57	30	10
Wheat tortilla (Mexican)	30	50	8
White wheat flour bread, average	70 ± 0	30	10

Food	Glycemic index (glucose = 100)	Serving size, g	Glycemic load per serving
Whole-meal rye bread (Canada)	58 ± 6	30	8
Whole-meal (whole-wheat) wheat-flour bread, average	71 ± 2	30	9
Wonder, enriched white bread, average	73 ± 2	30	10
BEVERAGES			
Apple juice, unsweetened, average	40 ± 1	250 ml	12
Carrot juice, freshly made (Sydney, Australia)	43 ± 3	250 ml	10
Cranberry juice cocktail (Ocean Spray Inc, Lakeville-Middleboro, MA, USA)	68 ± 3	250 ml	24
Orange juice, unsweetened, average	50 ± 4	250 ml	13
Pineapple juice, unsweetened (Dole Packaged Foods, Toronto, Canada)	46	250 ml	16
Tomato juice, canned, no added sugar (Berri Ltd, Berri, Australia)	38 ± 4	250 ml	4
BREAKFAST CEREALS AND RELATED PRODUCTS			
All-Bran (Kellogg's Inc, Canada)	51 ± 5	30	9
Cornflakes, average	81 ± 3	30	21
Cream of Wheat (Nabisco Brands Ltd, Canada)	66	250	17
Cream of Wheat, Instant (Nabisco Brands Ltd, Canada)	74	250	22
Life (Quaker Oats Co, Canada)	66	30	15
Muesli, NS (Canada)	66 ± 9	30	17
Muesli, No Name (Sunfresh Ltd, Toronto, Canada)	60	30	11

Food	Glycemic index (glucose = 100)	Serving size, g	Glycemic load per serving
Oat bran, raw (Quaker Oats Co, Canada)	50	10	2
Quick Oats, average	66 ± 1	250	17
Puffed Wheat (Quaker Oats Co, Canada)	67	30	17
Rice Krispies (Kellogg's Inc, Canada)	82	30	22
Raisin Bran (Kellogg's, USA)	61 ± 5	30	12
Special K (Kellogg's, USA)	69 ± 5	30	14
GRAINS			
Barley pearled, average	25 ± 1	150	11
Bulgur, boiled (Canada)	48 ± 2	150	12
Couscous, boiled 5 min, average	65 ± 4	150	23
Corn sweet, average	53 ± 4	150	17
Rice: long grain, white, boiled 7 min (Star brand; Gouda foods, Concord, Canada)	64 ± 3	150	26
Rice: brown (Canada)	66 ± 5	150	21
Rice: instant, white, boiled 1 min (Canada)	46	150	19
Whole wheat kernels, average	41 ± 3	50 (dry)	14
DAIRY PRODUCTS			
Milk, full fat, average	27 ± 4	250 ml	3
Milk, skim (Canada)	32 ± 5	250 ml	4
Yogurt, NS (Canada)	36 ± 4	200	3
Yogurt: low-fat, fruit, sugar (Ski; Dairy Farmers, Australia)	33 ± 7	200	10

Food	Glycemic index (glucose = 100)	Serving size, g	Glycemic load per serving
Yogurt: nonfat, sweetened with acesulfame K and Splenda. Diet Vaalia, strawberry (Pauls Ltd, Australia)	23 ± 2	200	3
RAW FRUITS			
Apple, average	38 ± 2	120	6
Apricots, NS (Italy)	57	120	5
Banana, ripe, all yellow (USA)	51	120	13
Banana, slightly underripe, yellow with green sections (USA)	42	120	11
Banana, overripe, yellow flecked with brown (USA)	48	120	12
Cherries, NS (Canada)	22	120	3
Grapefruit, (Canada)	25	120	3
Grapes, average	46 ± 3	120	8
Kiwi, average	53 ± 6	120	6
Mango, average	51 ± 5	120	8
Orange, average	42 ± 3	120	5
Peach, average	42 ± 14	120	5
Pear, average	38 ± 2	120	4
Pineapple, average	59 ± 8	120	7
Plum, average	39 ± 15	120	5
Rockmelon/Cantaloupe, (Australia)	65 ± 9	120	4
Strawberries (Australia)	40 ± 7	120	1
Watermelon (Australia)	72 ± 13	120	4

Food	Glycemic index (glucose = 100)	Serving size, g	Glycemic load per serving
CANNED FRUITS			
Apricots, canned in light syrup (Riviera, Aliments Caneast Foods, Montreal, Canada)	64	120	12
Fruit Cocktail, canned (Delmonte Canadian Canners Ltd, Hamilton, Canada)	55	120	9
Peach, canned in natural juice, average	38 ± 8	120	4
Peach, canned in light syrup (Delmonte, Canadian Canners Ltd)	52	120	9
Pear, canned in pear juice, Bartlett (Delmonte Canadian Canners Ltd)	44	120	5
DRIED FRUITS			
Apple (Australia)	29 ± 5	60	10
Apricots, average	31 ± 1	60	9
Dates (Australia)	103 ± 21	60	42
Figs, tenderized, Dessert Maid brand (Ernest Hall andSons, Sydney, Australia)	61 ± 6	60	16
Prunes, pitted (Sunsweet Growers Inc., Yuba City, CA, USA)	29 ± 4	60	10
Raisin (Canada)	64 ± 11	60	28
BEANS			
Baked beans, average	48 ± 8	150	7
Beans, dried, boiled	29 ± 9	150	9
Chickpeas, average	28 ± 6	150	8
Haricot and navy beans, dried, boiled (Canada)	30	150	9

Food	Glycemic index (glucose = 100)	Serving size, g	Glycemic load per serving
Haricot and navy beans, boiled (Canada)	31 ± 6	150	9
Kidney beans, canned (Lancia-Bravo Foods Ltd, Canada)	52	150	9
Lentils, green, dried, boiled, average	30 ± 4	150	5
Lentils, red, dried, boiled, average	26 ± 4	150	5
Peas, dried, boiled (Australia)	22	150	2
NUTS			
Cashew nuts, salted (Coles Supermarkets, Australia	22 ± 5	50	3
Peanuts, average	14 ± 8	50	1
PASTA and NOODLES			
Instant noodles, average	47 ± 1	180	19
Macaroni, average	47 ± 2	180	23
Macaroni and cheese, boxed (Kraft General Foods Canada Inc, Don Mills, Canada)	64	180	32
Spaghetti, white, boiled 5 min, average	38 ± 3	180	18
Tortellini, cheese (Stouffer; Nestlé, Don Mills, Canada)	50	180	10
VEGETABLES			
Beetroot (Canada)	64 ± 16	80	5
Baked potato Ontario, white, baked in skin (Canada)	60	150	18
Boiled potato, Ontario, white, peeled, cut into cubes, boiled in salted water 15 min (Canada)	58	150	16

Food	Glycemic index (glucose = 100)	Serving size, g	Glycemic load per serving
Carrots, average	47 ± 16	80	3
Green peas, average	48 ± 5	80	3
Sweet corn, average	54 ± 4	80	9
Sweet potato, average	61 ± 7	150	17
MISCELLANEOUS			
Hummus (chickpea salad dip)	6 ± 4	30	0
Honey, average	55 ± 5	25	10
Popcorn, plain, cooked in microwave oven, average	72 ± 17	20	8

APPENDIX 3

Smart Food Swaps
(American Heart Association Inc, n.d.-a; Lillis, 2019)

Instead of this	Eat this
BAKERY PRODUCTS AND BREAD	
Bread and rolls	Bowl of steel-cut oats
Burritos and tacos	Whole-grain tortillas
White bread	Grains: barley, brown rice, quinoa Whole-grain bread
BEVERAGES	
Soda, soft or sugary drinks, juice	Compote from frozen fruits (without sugar) Homemade smoothies Water Water with lemon or mint or berries

Instead of this	Eat this
BEANS	
Canned beans	Cook dry beans or at least rinse canned with water several times
BREAKFAST CEREALS AND RELATED PRODUCTS	
Cornflakes	Bran flakes
Instant oatmeal	Steel-cut oats
Sugary cereal	Cereal with less amount of sugar
DAIRY PRODUCTS	
Sweet, flavored yogurt	Plain or Greek yogurt with fresh or frozen fruits
Ice cream	Homemade fruit popsicles
DESSERTS	
Chocolate spreads like Nutella	Peanut butter
Chocolate bar	Homemade "ice cream" from the frozen banana and cocoa powder

Instead of this	Eat this
Desserts and sweets	Fresh, frozen fruits
Jelly, jam	Fresh strawberries
Store-bought granola	Banana Homemade granola with nuts and seeds
FRUITS	
Banana, ripe	Banana, green
Dry fruits	Fresh fruits Frozen fruits
Canned fruits in syrup	Fresh, frozen fruits
GRAINS	
Corn	Peas Leafy greens
White rice	Brown rice Converted rice

Instead of this	Eat this
MISCELLANEOUS	
Store-bought sauces, ketchup, dressing	Homemade sauces without sugar
Sugar or honey for baking	Banana, cinnamon
Commercially prepared popcorn	Homemade air-popped popcorn
Canned soup	Homemade soup
Frozen pizza	Homemade pizza with homemade sauce, fresh vegetables, and light cheese
PASTA AND NOODLES	
Macaroni and spaghetti	Brown rice Quinoa Vegetable's spaghetti
VEGETABLES	
Baked potato	Bulgur
Cooked vegetables	Raw vegetables (when possible)

REFERENCES

Ahola, A. J., Mutter, S., Forsblom, C., Harjutsalo, V., & Groop, P.-H. (2019). *Meal timing, meal frequency, and breakfast skipping in adult individuals with type 1 diabetes – associations with glycaemic control. Scientific Reports, 9(1).* https://doi.org/10.1038/s41598-019-56541-5 This article is published under Creative Commons — Attribution 4.0 International license (CC BY 4.0) https://creativecommons.org/licenses/by/4.0/

American Heart Association Inc. (n.d.-a). *Rethink Your Drink Guidebook.* https://www.heart.org/-/media/files/affiliates/wsa/oregon/oregon-rethink-your-drink-guidebook.pdf

American Heart Association Inc. (n.d.-b). *Sugar Recom-*

mendation Healthy Kids and Teens Infographic. https://
www.heart.org/en/healthy-living/healthy-eating/eat-
smart/sugar/sugar-recommendation-healthy-kids-
and-teens-infographic#:~:text=Healthy%20Kids%
20are%20Sweet%20Enough

American Heart Association Inc. (2017, April 17). *Sugar
101.* https://www.heart.org/en/healthy-living/healthy-
eating/eat-smart/sugar/sugar-101#:~:text=Naturally%
20occurring%20sugars%20are%20found

American Heart Association Inc. (2019). *How much
sugar is too much?* American Heart Association. https://
www.heart.org/en/healthy-living/healthy-eating/eat-
smart/sugar/how-much-sugar-is-too-much

Brown West-Rosenthal, L. (2017, March 17). *16 Foods
That Stop Sugar Cravings.* Eat This Not That. https://
www.eatthis.com/stop-sugar-cravings/

Calihan, J. (2021, November 19). *21 high-protein snacks,
ranked.* DietDoctor. https://www.dietdoctor.com/high-
protein/snacks
Adapted and reproduced by permission of DietDoctor

Chichger H., (2018, March 19) *Artificial sweeteners may
make you fat.* The Conversation. https://theconversa

tion.com/artificial-sweeteners-may-make-you-fat-93452
This article is published under Creative Commons — Attribution/No derivatives license. Attribution-NoDerivatives 4.0 International (CC BY-ND 4.0) https://creativecommons.org/licenses/by-nd/4.0/

Cleveland Clinic. (2020a, April 3). *Do You Really Need to Eat Breakfast?* Health Essentials from Cleveland Clinic. https://health.clevelandclinic.org/do-you-really-need-to-eat-breakfast/

Cleveland Clinic. (2020b, August 7). *The Whole Truth About Whole Grains.* Health Essentials from Cleveland Clinic. https://health.clevelandclinic.org/the-whole-truth-about-whole-grains/

Confucius (551-479 B.C.). Public Domain.

Conner A., & Brown J. (2018, April 23) *Artificial sweeteners linked to diabetes and obesity.* The Conversation. https://theconversation.com/artificial-sweeteners-linked-to-diabetes-and-obesity-95314
This article is published under Creative Commons — Attribution/No derivatives license. Attribution-NoDerivatives 4.0 International (CC BY-ND 4.0) https://creativecommons.org/licenses/by-nd/4.0/

Diabetes Food Hub. (2020, February). *What is the Diabetes Plate Method?* Diabetes Food Hub. https://www.diabetesfoodhub.org/articles/what-is-the-diabetes-plate-method.html
Reprinted with permission from The American Diabetes Association. Copyright 2021 by the American Diabetes Association

Fisher, L. (2020, January). *5 Ways to Boost Energy Without Sugar or Coffee.* Real Simple. https://www.realsimple.com/food-recipes/recipe-collections-favorites/healthy-meals/how-to-boost-energy

Fletcher, J. (2020, December 22). *Bedtime snacks for diabetes: Which foods are best and why?* Www.medical-newstoday.com. https://www.medicalnewstoday.com/articles/324881#glucose-levels
Republished from "Bedtime snacks for diabetes: Which foods are best and why?" by Fletcher, J. by permission of Medical News Today.

Foster-Powell, K., Holt, S. H., & Brand-Miller, J. C. (2002). *International table of glycemic index and glycemic load values: 2002. The American Journal of Clinical Nutrition, 76(1),* 5–56. https://doi.org/10.1093/ajcn/76.1.5
Adapted and reproduced by permission of Oxford

University Press on behalf of the American Society for
Nutrition.

Gameau, D. (2015, March). *Added Sugar VS Natural
Sugar, How Much Natural Sugar Per Day*. That Sugar
Movement, https://thatsugarmovement.com/added-
sugar-vs-natural-sugar/

Gearing, M. E. (2015, October 5). *Natural and Added
Sugars: Two Sides of the Same Coin*. Science in the News.
https://sitn.hms.harvard.edu/flash/2015/natural-and-
added-sugars-two-sides-of-the-same-coin/

Harvard School of Public Health. (2012, September 18).
How Sweet Is It? https://www.hsph.harvard.edu/nutri
tionsource/healthy-drinks/sugary-drinks/how-sweet-
is-it/

Harvard School of Public Health. (2013, August 5).
Added Sugar in the Diet. The Nutrition Source. https://
www.hsph.harvard.edu/nutritionsource/carbohy
drates/added-sugar-in-the-diet/#ref27

Hyman, M. (2014, May 26). *5 Reasons Most Diets Fail (and
How To Succeed)*. Dr. Mark Hyman. https://drhyman.
com/blog/2014/05/26/5-reasons-diets-fail-succeed/

Kandola, A. (2019a, January 9). *Most effective fat-burning foods for weight loss*. Www.medicalnewstoday.com. https://www.medicalnewstoday.com/articles/324130
Republished from "Most effective fat-burning foods for weight loss" by Kandola, A. by permission of Medical News Today.

Kandola, A. (2019b, January 9). *The 5 best nuts for diabetes*. Www.medicalnewstoday.com. https://www.medicalnewstoday.com/articles/324141#why-are-nuts-useful-for-diabetes
Republished from "The 5 best nuts for diabetes" by Kandola, A. by permission of Medical News Today.

Lillis, C. (2019, March 12). *How to reduce sugar intake.* Www.medicalnewstoday.com. https://www.medicalnewstoday.com/articles/324673#how-to-reduce-intake
Republished from "How to reduce sugar intake?" by Lillis, C. by permission of Medical News Today.

Link, R. (2019, January 19). *The Seeds that Support Weight Loss, Blood Sugar & More*. Dr. Axe. https://draxe.com/nutrition/caraway-seeds/

Live Naturally Magazine. (2013, March 14). *7 Foods*

That Fill You Up. Live Naturally Magazine. https://live
naturallymagazine.com/7-foods-that-fill-you-up/

Mad'a, P. (2016). *8. Limbic System • Functions of Cells and
Human Body*. Functions of Cells and Human Body
Multimedia Textbook. http://fblt.cz/en/skripta/regu
lacni-mechanismy-2-nervova-regulace/9-limbicky-
system/#:~:text=If%20we%20stimulate%20some%
20parts

Mad About Berries. (2020, July 19). *Glycemic Index and
Glycemic Load of Common Berries and Other Foods*. Mad
about Berries. https://www.madaboutberries.com/arti
cles/glycemic-index-and-glycemic-load.html

Mayo Clinic. (2018, January 19). *Tips for drinking more
water*. Mayo Clinic Health System. https://www.
mayoclinichealthsystem.org/hometown-health/speak
ing-of-health/tips-for-drinking-more-water
Used with permission of Mayo Foundation for Medical
Education and Research, all rights reserved.

Mayo Clinic. (2020a, August 25). *Glycemic index diet:
What's behind the claims* Mayo Clinic. https://www.
mayoclinic.org/healthy-lifestyle/nutrition-and-
healthy-eating/in-depth/glycemic-index-diet/art-
20048478

Used with permission of Mayo Foundation for Medical Education and Research, all rights reserved.

Mayo Clinic. (2020b, October 14). *Water: How much should you drink every day?* Mayo Clinic. https://www. mayoclinic.org/healthy-lifestyle/nutrition-and-healthy-eating/in-depth/water/art-20044256#:~:text= So%20how%20much%20fluid%20does
Used with permission of Mayo Foundation for Medical Education and Research, all rights reserved.

Neal, S. (2020, February 22). *Healthy Alternatives to Sugary Drinks |.* Susanuneal.com. https://susanuneal. com/healthy-alternatives-to-sugary-drinks

Nolin K., (2022, January 05) *What's the difference between sugar, other natural sweeteners and artificial sweeteners? A food chemist explains sweet science.* The Conversation. https://theconversation.com/whats-the-difference-between-sugar-other-natural-sweeteners-and-artifi cial-sweeteners-a-food-chemist-explains-sweet-science-172571
This article is published under Creative Commons — Attribution/No derivatives license. Attribution-NoDerivatives 4.0 International (CC BY-ND 4.0) https://creativecommons.org/licenses/by-nd/4.0/

Patrick, C. (2020, May 12). *Gratitude - a mindset for weight loss*. FastFx | Meal Replacement Designed by Gastroenterologists. https://www.fastfx.co.nz/grati tude-a-mindset-for-weight-loss/

Piper, W. Illustrated by Hauman, G. & Hauman, D. (2000). *The Little Engine that Could (complete original edition)*. Platt & Munk, Publishers, a division of Grosset & Dunlap, Inc.

Randolph, K. (2002, May 12). *Sports Visualizations*. Llewellyn.com. https://www.llewellyn.com/encyclope dia/article/244
COPYRIGHT (2002) Llewellyn Worldwide, Ltd. All rights reserved.

Reichelt A., (2019, November 14) *Your brain on sugar: What the science actually says*. The Conversation. https:// theconversation.com/your-brain-on-sugar-what-the-science-actually-says-126581
This article is published under Creative Commons — Attribution/No derivatives license. Attribution-NoDerivatives 4.0 International (CC BY-ND 4.0) https://creativecommons.org/licenses/by-nd/4.0/

Roman, J. (2018, August 13). *Seven stages of sugar with-drawal (And why it's all worth it!)*. Dr. Alan Macdonald,

Dentist. http://dralanmacdonald.com/seven-stages-of-sugar-withdrawal-and-why-its-all-worth-it/

Santos-Longhurst, A. (2020, July 28). *What Is a Sugar Detox? Effects and How to Avoid Sugar.* Healthline. https://www.healthline.com/health/sugar-detox-symptoms

Schwenk, D. (2018, October 7). *Does Your Gut Help Control Food Cravings?* Cultured Food Life. https://www.culturedfoodlife.com/does-your-gut-help-control-food-cravings/

Serrano, I. (2021, January 15). *How to Use the Power of the Mind to Reduce Sugar Intake.* [Personal communication].

Smith, C. (2020). *Zero sugar detox. Discover how you can overcome your silent addiction, crush your cravings, and burn fat effortlessly in the process.* Nealco Press.

Spritzler, F. (2021a, October 04). *The truth about "fat-burning foods".* DietDoctor. https://www.dietdoctor.com/weight-loss/fat-burning-foods
Adapted and reproduced by permission of DietDoctor.

Spritzler, F. (2021b, December 14). *The best high-protein*

foods for weight loss. DietDoctor. https://www.dietdoc
tor.com/high-protein/foods
Adapted and reproduced by permission of DietDoctor

Story, M., & French, S. (2004). *Food Advertising and
Marketing Directed at Children and Adolescents in the US*.
International Journal of Behavioral Nutrition and
Physical Activity, 1(1), 3. https://doi.org/10.1186/
1479-5868-1-3
This article is published under Creative Commons —
Attribution 4.0 International license (CC BY 4.0)
https://creativecommons.org/licenses/by/4.0/

Sukel, K. (2019, August 1). *What Happens at The Synapse?*
Dana Foundation. https://dana.org/article/qa-neuro
transmission-the-synapse/#:~:text=The%20synapse%
2C%20rather%2C%20is%20that

Thomas, P. (2020, May 4). *How to use Lofty Questions to
Transform Your Life*. Self Help for Life. https://selfhelp
forlife.com/lofty-questions/

Tocino-Smith, J. (2019, July 4). *What is Locke's Goal
Setting Theory of Motivation? (Incl. Examples)*. Positive-
Psychology.com. https://positivepsychology.com/goal-
setting-theory/

Union of Concerned Scientists. (2016, May). *Sugar-Coating Science*. Www.ucsusa.org. https://www.ucsusa.org/resources/sugar-coating-science

U.S. Department of Agriculture and U.S. Department of Health and Human Services. (2020, December). *Dietary Guidelines for Americans, 2020-2025. 9th Edition.* https://www.dietaryguidelines.gov/resources/2020-2025-dietary-guidelines-online-materials
The information presented on DietaryGuidelines.gov website is considered public domain information. This means it may be freely distributed and copied — but please include a link to our website and acknowledge USDA and HHS as the source.

U.S. Food & Drug Administration. (2020a, March 10). *Added Sugars on the New Nutrition Facts Label.* FDA. https://www.fda.gov/food/new-nutrition-facts-label/added-sugars-new-nutrition-facts-label

U.S. Food & Drug Administration. (2020b). *How to Understand and Use the Nutrition Facts Label.* FDA. https://www.fda.gov/food/new-nutrition-facts-label/how-understand-and-use-nutrition-facts-label

U.S. Food & Drug Administration. (2021). *Changes to the Nutrition Facts Label.* FDA. https://www.fda.gov/food/

food-labeling-nutrition/changes-nutrition-facts-label#:
~:text=Manufacturers%20with%20%2410%
20million%20or

Willard, C. (2019, January 17). *6 Ways to Practice Mindful Eating - Mindful* Mindful. https://www.mindful.org/6
ways-practice-mindful-eating/

Williams, L. (n.d.). *Reading: Expectancy Theory | Introduction to Business.* Courses.lumenlearning.com. https://
courses.lumenlearning.com/wmintrobusiness/chapter/
reading-expectancy-theory/#:~:text=Expectancy%
20is%20the%20individual
This article is published under Creative Commons —
Attribution-ShareAlike 4.0 International licence (CC
BY-SA 4.0) https://creativecommons.org/licenses/
by/4.0/

Printed in Great Britain
by Amazon

83762803R00139